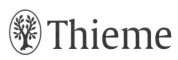

Practical Guides in Interventional Radiology

Varicose Veins

Felipe B. Collares, MD, MSc, RVS
Director
Massachusetts Vein Care Center and Vascular Ultrasound
Interventional Radiologist
Beth Israel Deaconess Medical Center
Instructor
Harvard Medical School
Boston, Massachusetts

Salomão Faintuch, MD, MSc
Editor and Series Editor
Clinical Director of Interventional Radiology
Beth Israel Deaconess Medical Center
Assistant Professor
Harvard Medical School
Boston, Massachusetts

Thieme
New York • Stuttgart • Delhi • Rio de Janeiro

Executive Editor: William Lamsback
Managing Editor: Elizabeth Palumbo
Director, Editorial Services: Mary Jo Casey
Assistant Managing Editor: Haley Paskalides
Production Editor: Sean Woznicki
International Production Director: Andreas Schabert
International Marketing Director: Fiona Henderson
International Sales Director: Louisa Turrell
Director of Sales, North America: Mike Roseman
Senior Vice President and Chief Operating Officer:
  Sarah Vanderbilt
President: Brian D. Scanlan

Library of Congress Cataloging-in-Publication Data

Names: Collares, Felipe, editor. | Faintuch, Salomão, editor.
Title: Practical Guides in Interventional Radiology: Varicose
  veins / [edited by] Felipe Collares, Salomão Faintuch.
Other titles: Varicose veins (Faintuch) | Practical guides in
  interventional radiology.
Description: New York : Thieme, [2017] | Series: Practical
  guides in interventional radiology series | Includes bib-
  liographical references.
Identifiers: LCCN 2017005195| ISBN 9781626230125 (print)
  | ISBN 9781626230132 (e-book)
Subjects: | MESH: Varicose Veins–therapy | Varicose
  Veins–diagnosis |
  Endovascular Procedures | Ambulatory Care Classification:
  LCC RC695 | NLM WG 620 | DDC 616.1/43–dc23
LC record available at https://lccn.loc.gov/2017005195

© 2017 Thieme Medical Publishers, Inc.

Thieme Publishers New York
333 Seventh Avenue, New York, NY 10001 USA
+1 800 782 3488, customerservice@thieme.com

Thieme Publishers Stuttgart
Rüdigerstrasse 14, 70469 Stuttgart, Germany
+49 [0]711 8931 421, customerservice@thieme.de

Thieme Publishers Delhi
A-12, Second Floor, Sector-2, Noida-201301
Uttar Pradesh, India
+91 120 45 566 00, customerservice@thieme.in

Thieme Publishers Rio de Janeiro, Thieme Publicações Ltda.
Edifício Rodolpho de Paoli, 25º andar
Av. Nilo Peçanha, 50 – Sala 2508
Rio de Janeiro 20020-906 Brasil
+55 21 3172 2297 / +55 21 3172-1896

Cover design: Thieme Publishing Group
Typesetting by DiTech Processing Solutions

Printed in India by Replika Press Pvt Ltd   5 4 3 2 1
ISBN 978-1-62623-012-5

Also available as an e-book:
eISBN 978-1-62623-013-2

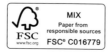

To my parents for their unconditional love and support throughout my life and to my brother for our cherished childhood memories and friendship. To my wife Juliana, who moved from the other side of the planet to be with me, changed my world for the better, and showed me the meaning of unconditional love by giving me our children Eduardo and Rafael.

Felipe B. Collares

To the Creator, Tammy, David, Jonathan, Rachel, Papai, and Mamãe. Everything I have achieved and will ever achieve in life is because of you and dedicated to you. If I were to explain here how much I owe you and appreciate you, there would be very few pages left to discuss Varicose Veins.

Salomão Faintuch

Contents

Foreword

Varicose Veins: Outpatient Interventional Series is a complete, well-illustrated, and easily understandable textbook on varicose veins and their current management.

The first two chapters review anatomy and pathophysiology. The overall anatomy of the superficial venous system is clearly presented as well as the histologic difference between arteries and veins. This chapter lays the anatomic groundwork for the management of pathology of the superficial venous system.

The physiology and pathophysiology of the venous system is then succinctly reviewed, integrating both the superficial and deep venous components. The physiology of normal venous return is hemodynamically explained, serving as the basis for the subsequent pathology of venous valvular incompetence at the various anatomic levels.

The initial patient-physician interaction is well covered in the chapter on the Clinical Exam. The authors generously include their Initial Visit Questionnaire for others to use, or it can serve as a foundation for a revised version for individual practices. Objective documentation of the physical findings, appropriate use of the CEAP classification, the Venous Clinical Severity Score, and the CVIQ-20 QOL questionnaire are reviewed. This overview serves as a model of how the patient's presentation should be memorialized in the medical record. The authors also review the advantages of photographic documentation in the medical record. This chapter is appropriately concluded with a discussion of managing patient expectations and establishing realistic goals for treatment.

The importance of imaging the venous system is covered in Chapter 4. Venous duplex is the pertinent technique with all of the important points covered with good quality images serving as examples. This chapter is a "how-to" guide for the performance of a good venous duplex examination.

The remainder of the text is devoted to treatment. Appropriately, the first therapy discussed is compression. After a brief review of the causes of edema via the venous and lymphatic circulation, the various types of and indications for compression are discussed.

Thermal ablation is the most commonly used technique to eliminate pathologic reflux in the superficial system. A clearly descriptive and pictoral review is covered in Chapter 6.

Sclerotherapy, which is increasing in popularity, is covered nicely in Chapter 7. The variety of sclerosants and their proper application are put into clear perspective. The chapter concludes with how to recognize and avoid complications of sclerotherapy.

The technique of ambulatory phlebectomy is well reviewed in Chapter 8. The authors offer a step-by-step guide to performing procedures and managing the patient post procedure.

Perhaps one of the most helpful chapters, especially for those new to the field, is Chapter 9, which covers Safety, Quality, and Complications. This review helps with risk assessment, decision making, recognizing, and treating the spectrum of complications.

The text appropriately concludes with a discussion of New Endovascular Techniques, focusing on microfoam, cyanoacrylate glue, and mechanical-chemical ablation.

In summary, this text is of value for all practitioners managing superficial venous disease. It is especially valuable for the younger, less experienced practitioners.

The authors are congratulated for putting together this practical, concise, and well-illustrated text on varicose veins.

Anthony J. Comerota, MD FACS, FACC
Adjunct Professor of Surgery
University of Michigan
Ann Arbor, Michigan

Series Preface

For decades, practitioners have used classic textbooks of several thousand pages to study Interventional Radiology and Vascular Surgery. We, however, identified a great need for small, subject-focused, and clinically oriented guides to help practitioners and trainees master key skills on the job. We envisioned both portable printed books that could be easily carried to the clinic, procedure suite, and inpatient ward, as well as new technologies accessible on any phone, tablet, or computer. This Practical Guides in Interventional Radiology Series is extremely valuable for residents, fellows, practicing physicians, and mid-level practitioners who are currently involved in or look forward to specializing in the interventional radiology spectrum. Book chapters systematically cover indications, contraindications, patient selection and preprocedure workup, procedural technique, postprocedure management and follow-up, side effects and complications, clinical data and outcomes, and key references.

Varicose veins has been an area of tremendous growth and interest over the last 20 years, with a large paradigm shift from older surgical techniques to minimally invasive endovascular and injectable therapies.

I am very pleased to see that the entire spectrum of minimally invasive therapies for varicose veins are so well represented in our Varicose Veins volume. Our lead editor, Felipe Birchal Collares, MD, MSc of Beth Israel Deaconess Medical Center, Harvard Medical School and Mass Vein Care Center, did a wonderful job working with a stellar group of authors from across the nation and beyond. His many years of expertise in the treatment of varicose veins, together with his involvement and leadership in the American College of Phlebology helped to create a very useful guide for Interventional Radiologists, Vascular Surgeons, Dermatologists and other specialists interested in the treatment of varicose veins.

We hope that readers find our new Practical Guides in Interventional Radiology Series to be a more value-added way to master procedures and clinical care skills in a more focused and time-efficient manner.

Salomão Faintuch, MD, MSc
Series Editor, Practical Guides in Interventional
Radiology

Preface

One in four adults in this country has varicose veins. If spider and reticular veins are included, the prevalence increases to above 80% of the population. Out of these millions of people, many seek treatment due to disease-related symptoms or for cosmetic reasons, while others should seek treatment due to the associated risk of chronic venous insufficiency, including severe skin changes and ulcers.

The cause of such a highly prevalent and undertreated spectrum of diseases should draw the attention and interest of Interventional Radiologists, Vascular Surgeons and Vascular Medicine specialists. Patients suffering from venous insufficiency need our help and the current available treatment options are efficient in improving their symptoms and overall quality of life significantly.

While vein stripping and traditional surgery has been used for more than a century, these treatments have been largely replaced by percutaneous and minimally invasive endovascular therapies due to their high efficacy, safety, tolerability and the ability to be performed in the ambulatory office.

This textbook has been designed to bring both trainees and practitioners to the level of knowledge and expertise necessary to evaluate and treat their patients with minimally invasive endovascular treatments (including thermal and sclerosant-based modalities) which are continuously evolving, as we try to make them faster and more easily tolerated. Here we cover relevant anatomy and pathophysiology; clinical exam and imaging evaluation; compression, thermal and sclerosant therapies; ambulatory phlebectomy; quality and safety; and new non-thermal endovascular treatment options.

A great team of physicians from our Harvard hospitals, together with key national and international specialists have done a superb job providing comprehensive, yet concise, coverage of the full spectrum of current therapies, plus some insight into future therapies coming down the pipeline.

We believe it is time for all interventional and vascular specialists to become experts in varicose veins, and this book is a great, high-yield resource to achieve it in a timely and efficient manner.

Felipe B. Collares
Salomão Faintuch

Contributors

Edward H. Ahn, MD
Interventional Radiologist
Advanced Radiology
Baltimore, Maryland

Cyrillo R. Araujo, Jr., MD
Associate Professor in Radiology (tenured)
Director of Ultrasound
Radiology Quality and Safety Officer
University of Mississippi Medical Center
Jackson, Mississippi

Ian M. Brennan, MD
Interventional Radiologist
St. James's Hospital
Dublin, Ireland

Ann L. Brown, MD
Assistant Professor of Radiology
University of Cincinnati
Cincinnati, Ohio

Carlos Alberto M. Carvalho, MD
Vascular Surgeon and Phlebologist
President
Brazilian Association of Phlebology and Lymphology
President and Director
Clinical Laser VariMedical
Santos, Brazil

Felipe B. Collares, MD, MSc, RVS
Director
Massachusetts Vein Care Center and Vascular
    Ultrasound
Interventional Radiologist
Beth Israel Deaconess Medical Center
Instructor in Radiology
Harvard Medical School
Boston, Massachusetts

Amy R. Deipolyi, MD, PhD
Assistant Professor and Attending Physician
Interventional Radiology
Memorial Sloan Kettering Cancer Center
New York, New York

Salomão Faintuch, MD, MSc
Clinical Director of Interventional Radiology
Beth Israel Deaconess Medical Center
Assistant Professor of Radiology
Harvard Medical School
Boston, Massachusetts

Lauren Ferrara, MD
Interventional Radiology Fellow
Brigham and Women's Hospital
Boston, Massachusetts

Suvranu Ganguli, MD
Assistant Professor of Radiology
Harvard Medical School
Staff Radiologist
Vascular and Interventional Radiology
Massachusetts General Hospital
Boston, Massachusetts

Erica A. Gupta, MD
Diagnostic Radiologist
MetroWest Radiology Associates
Framingham, Massachusetts

Michael G. Johnson Jr., MD
Interventional Radiologist & Medical Director
Middletown Vein and Aesthetic Center
Attending Interventional Radiologist
Middlesex Hospital
Middletown, Conneticut

Indravadan J. Patel, MD
Assistant Professor
Vascular and Interventional Radiology
University Hospitals Case Medical Center
Cleveland, Ohio

Gloria M. Martinez Salazar, MD
Radiologist
Division of Interventional Radiology
Massachusetts General Hospital
Assistant Professor of Radiology
Harvard Medical School
Boston, Massachusetts

Igor Rafael Sincos, MD, PhD, MBA
Clinical Endovascular SP
Albert Einstein Hospital
São Paulo, Brazil

Raphael J. Yoo, MD, MS
Adult and Pediatric Vascular and Interventional
  Radiologist
Texas Children's Hospital/Baylor College of Medicine
Houston, Texas

1 Anatomy

Felipe B. Collares

1.1 Introduction

Anatomic knowledge is the foundation of clinical phlebology, being crucial for the management of venous disorders in the lower extremity. Our understanding of the morphology and pathophysiology of chronic venous insufficiency and varicose veins has significantly improved in recent years, which made the traditional anatomical nomenclature of the official *Terminologia Anatomica*[1] somewhat deficient. Accurate terminology of the veins in the lower limb became a challenge for phlebologists given that imprecise identification of veins in the lower limb remained an important source of confusion. The use of inaccurate nomenclature can make the exchange of information in clinical literature difficult and lead to inappropriate management of venous diseases. For instance, the "superficial femoral vein," which is the main deep vein in the thigh, could be erroneously considered as a vessel of the superficial venous system[2] and abbreviations such as "LSV" could be interpreted as either the "long" or the "lesser" saphenous vein.[3] In addition, the indiscriminate use of eponyms that were not part of the official anatomic terminology could lead to further misconception and confusion. For this reason, in 2001, an International Interdisciplinary Committee was designated to revise the nomenclature of the lower extremity venous system and update the terminology where clinically relevant.[4,5] This consensus document, stimulated by the need for revision and extension of the *Terminologia Anatomica*, offered an internationally acceptable venous anatomic terminology for the lower extremity venous system, which is adequate for both anatomists and clinicians.

The terminology and definitions used in this textbook conform to the newest revision of the nomenclature. Therefore, discontinued names such as "superficial femoral vein," "long or greater saphenous vein," and "short or lesser saphenous vein" are replaced by their respective accurate terms: "femoral vein," "great saphenous vein," and "small saphenous vein," respectively. Eponyms are discouraged in publications and only a few well-known names that have been retained, such as "Giacomini's vein," are mentioned in this chapter. The official Latin terms are written in *italics*.

1.2 General Considerations

The venules are considered the first part of the venous system, and receive blood from the capillaries (▶ Fig. 1.1). These small vascular structures measure 20 μm in diameter, and consist of endothelial cells surrounded by collagen fibers. As the diameter of the venules increases, smooth muscle cells start to appear within the fibrous sheath, and at a diameter of 200 μm, the muscle layer becomes well defined. When the vessel achieves a clinically visible size, the vein is composed of three distinct layers: endothelial lining (*tunica intima*); smooth muscle cells (*tunica media*); and collagen fibers (*tunica adventitia*) (▶ Fig. 1.2). The composition of the vein wall is variable, and the muscular content

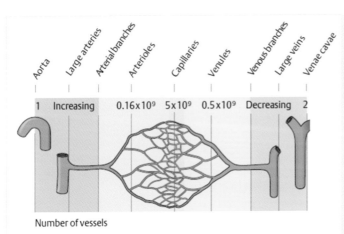

Aorta	Large arteries	Arterial branches	Arterioles	Capillaries	Venules	Venous branches	Large veins	Venae cavae

| 1 | Increasing | 0.16x10⁹ | 5x10⁹ | 0.5x10⁹ | Decreasing | 2 |

Number of vessels

Fig. 1.1 Scheme of the peripheral systemic circulation. (Reproduced with permission from Schuenke M, Schulte E, Schumacher U. General Anatomy and Musculoskeletal System. Stuttgart: Thieme; 2010. Illustration by Karl Wesker.)

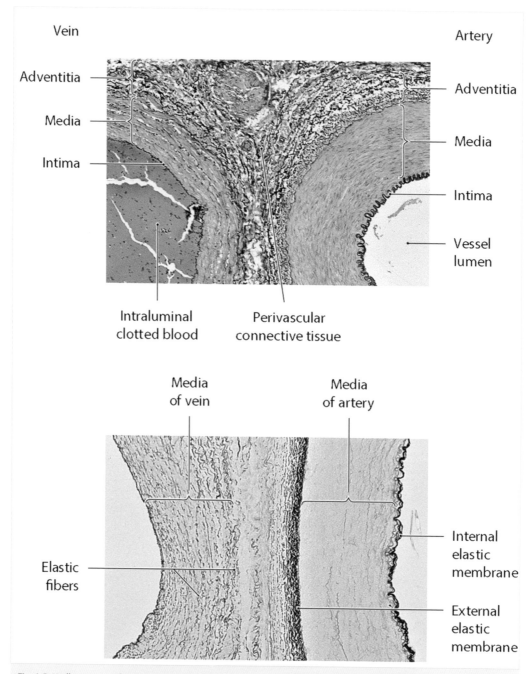

Fig. 1.2 Wall structure of arteries and veins. (Reproduced with permission from Schuenke M, Schulte E, Schumacher U. General Anatomy and Musculoskeletal System. Stuttgart: Thieme; 2010.)

of the media changes depending on the location and on the hydrostatic pressure of the vessel. Microscopic valves in small veins and venules consist of delicate connective tissue lined with endothelial cells; and valves in larger veins are composed of collagen and smooth muscle covered by endothelium.[6,7,8,9,10,11]

The anatomy of the lower extremity venous system is extremely variable. As a general rule, the veins of the lower limb are divided into three independent but interconnected systems: the deep venous system, the superficial venous system, and the perforating veins. The deep venous system is located below the muscular fascia, while the superficial venous system lies in the subcutaneous tissue between the muscle fascia and the dermis. The perforating veins are a communication between the superficial and deep venous systems, while communicating veins interconnect with other vessels within the same compartment.[4]

1.3 Deep Veins

The deep veins in the lower extremity are located within the deep compartment delineated by the muscle fascia, and accompany the corresponding arteries and their branches. They contain a large number of valves and are regularly doubled as high as the level of the popliteal vein.[12,13,14] The structure of the deep venous system of the lower extremity is presented in ▶ Fig. 1.3, with its nomenclature summarized in ▶ Table 1.1.

1.3.1 Deep Veins of the Foot

The deep veins of the foot are the medial plantar veins (*venae plantares mediales*), the lateral plantar veins (*venae plantares laterales*), the deep plantar venous arch (*arcus venosus plantaris profundus*), the deep plantar metatarsal veins (*venae metatarsales plantares profundae*), the deep dorsal metatarsal veins (*venae metartasales dorsales profundae*), the deep plantar digital veins (*venae digitales plantares profundae*), the deep dorsal digital veins (*venae digitales dorsales profundae*), and the pedal veins (*venae dorsales pedis*) (▶ Fig. 1.3). The deep plantar digital veins drain the plexuses on the plantar aspect of the toes, communicate with the deep dorsal digital veins, and join to form four deep plantar metatarsal veins running inside the metatarsal space. At the dorsal aspect of the foot, the deep dorsal digital veins and deep dorsal metatarsal veins are arranged in a similar manner. These plantar and dorsal metatarsal veins communicate and join to form the deep plantar venous arch and the pedal veins, respectively. The pedal veins run on both sides of the dorsalis pedis artery, together with the deep fibular nerve. Different from the veins of the leg and the thigh, the valves of veins of the foot are oriented to allow the blood flow from the deep to the superficial veins.[4,13]

1.3.2 Deep Veins of the Leg

The deep veins of the leg are: the posterior tibial veins (*venae tibiales posteriores*), the anterior tibial veins (*venae tibiales anteriores*), the fibular veins (*venae fibulares*), the genicular venous plexus (*plexus venosus genicularis*), the soleal veins (*venae soleales*), the gastrocnemius veins (*venae gastrocnemii*), and the popliteal vein (*vena poplitea*) (▶ Fig. 1.3). The posterior tibial veins accompany the posterior tibial artery and receive tributaries from the posterior group of calf muscles, the venous plexus inside the soleal muscle or soleal veins, the perforator veins, and the fibular vein. These veins contain from 8 to 19 valves. The anterior tibial veins are a proximal continuation of the pedal veins after passing under the inferior extensor retinaculum; they accompany the anterior tibial artery and merge with posterior tibial veins to form the popliteal vein. These veins contain from 8 to 11 valves. The fibular veins travel along the corresponding artery and receive tributaries from the soleal and perforator veins before draining into the posterior tibial vein in the proximal calf. These veins contain from 8 to 11 valves. The gastrocnemius veins are situated within the medial and lateral gastrocnemius muscles and often merge into a common trunk emptying directly into the popliteal vein just distal to the small saphenous vein opening or into the saphenopopliteal junction. The soleal veins are situated in a deeper plane and drain the soleal muscle into either the posterior tibial veins or the fibular veins. The genicular venous plexus, a complex system of interconnected vessels, collects blood from the knee region in the popliteal fossa into the popliteal vein. The popliteal vein ascends through the popliteal fossa receiving several tributaries as described earlier and becomes the femoral vein after passing the adductor hiatus within the insertion of the adductor magnus muscle. The popliteal vein contains from one to four valves and can be duplicated in 5 to 20% of the cases.[4,13,14,15,16]

1.3.3 Deep Veins of the Thigh

The deep veins of the thigh are the common femoral vein (*vena femoralis communis*), the femoral vein (*vena femoralis*), the profunda femoris vein (*vena profunda femoris*), the medial circumflex femoral veins (*venae circumflexae femoris mediales*), the lateral circumflex femoral veins (*venae circumflexae femoris laterales*), the deep femoral communicating veins (*venae comitantes arteriarum perforantium*), and the sciatic vein (*vena comitans*

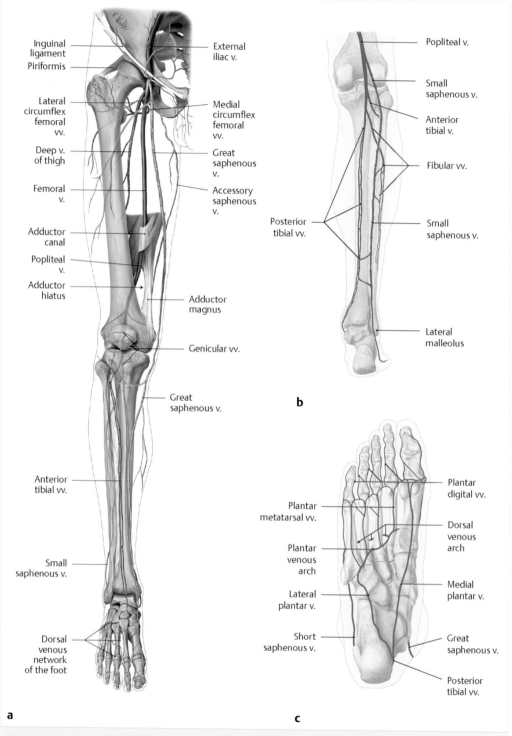

Fig. 1.3 Deep and superficial venous systems of the lower extremity. (Reproduced with permission from Gilroy AM, MacPherson BR, Ross LM, Schuenke M, Schulte E, Schumacher U. Atlas of Anatomy. 2nd ed. New York, NY: Thieme; 2012. Illustration by Karl Wesker and Marcus Voll.)

Table 1.1 Deep veins of the lower extremity

Nomenclature	Official Latin term
Medial plantar veins	*Venae plantares mediales*
Lateral plantar veins	*Venae plantares laterales*
Deep plantar venous arch	*Arcus venosus plantaris profundus*
Deep plantar metatarsal veins	*Venae metatarsales plantares profundae*
Deep dorsal metatarsal veins	*Venae metatarsales dorsales profundae*
Deep plantar digital veins	*Venae digitales plantares profundae*
Deep dorsal digital veins	*Venae digitales dorsales profundae*
Pedal veins	*Venae dorsales pedis*
Posterior tibial veins	*Venae tibiales posteriores*
Anterior tibial veins	*Venae tibiales anteriores*
Fibular veins	*Venae fibulares*
Genicular venous plexus	*Plexus venosus genicularis*
Soleal veins	*Venae soleales*
Gastrocnemius veins	*Venae gastrocnemii*
Popliteal vein	*Vena popliteal*
Common femoral vein	*Vena femoralis communis*
Femoral vein	*Vena femoralis*
Profunda femoris vein	*Vena profunda femoris*
Medial circumflex femoral veins	*Venae circumflexae femoris mediales*
Lateral circumflex femoral veins	*Venae circumflexae femoris laterales*
Deep femoral communicating veins	*Venae comitantes arteriarum perforantium*
Sciatic vein	*Vena comitans nervi ischiadici*

nervi ischiadici) (▶ Fig. 1.3). The femoral vein, previously named with the now unauthorized term "superficial femoral vein,"[2] originates at the superior margin of the popliteal fossa as a direct continuation of the popliteal vein. The vessel courses in the femoral canal and can appear duplicated in up to 46% of cases, isolated or in combination with popliteal vein duplications. Anatomic variations, duplications, and truncular venous malformations are frequently bilateral. The femoral vein usually contains from three to five valves.[13,14,17,18] The profunda femoris vein or deep femoral vein originates as a confluence of smaller muscular veins draining the posterior and lateral thigh and features several valves. The abandoned term "deep vein of the thigh" is nonspecific and misleading and should not be used.[4,13] The deep femoral communicating veins, formerly named "perforating veins," accompany the perforating arteries that originate from the deep femoral artery and pierce the adductor muscles to enter the posterior compartment of the thigh. The denomination "perforating," now reserved for veins that connect to both the superficial and deep venous systems, does not apply to these vessels because they never leave the deep compartment.[4,13] The medial and lateral circumflex femoral veins drain the thigh muscles and the hip joint frequently into the femoral vein or the common femoral vein, and rarely into the profunda femoris vein.[13] The common femoral vein originates from the confluence of the femoral vein and the profunda femoris vein which is usually situated from 1 to 3 cm distal to the femoral artery bifurcation or 4 to 12 cm distal to the inguinal ligament. The vein is situated within the iliopectineal fossa and becomes the external iliac vein, after passing under the inguinal ligament and entering the pelvis. It only contains one valve, the suprasaphenic valve, which is present in around 80% of cases, located proximally to the saphenous opening, and protects the lower extremity superficial venous system from the elevated intra-abdominal pressures.[4,13,14] In 2009, the term sciatic vein (*vena ischiadica*) was replaced by axial vein of the lower limb (*vena axialis membri inferioris*) in the *Terminologia Embryologica* to name the main trunk of the primordial deep venous system.[13] It is located in the posterior portion of the lower extremity following the course of the sciatic nerve, and may persist as an important collateral pathway for the femoral vein.[13,19] The complete form of the persistent sciatic vein (*vena comitans nervi ischiadici*) originates from the popliteal vein or tributaries, extends through the dorsal aspect of the thigh and buttock, and terminates into the internal iliac vein. There are two different variations from the complete form: the proximal persistent sciatic vein and the distal persistent sciatic vein. The proximal persistent sciatic vein originates from the posterior superior aspect of the thigh and continues into the pelvis; and the distal persistent sciatic vein originates in posterior inferior aspect of the thigh, terminating into the profunda femoris vein.[13,19]

1.4 Superficial Veins

The superficial veins of the lower extremity are located in the superficial compartment, within the subcutaneous tissue between the dermis and the muscular fascia. The two most important superficial veins are the great saphenous vein (*vena saphena magna*) and the small saphenous vein (*vena saphena parva*). In the consensus document of 2002, the terms "great" and "small" were chosen for the nomenclature of the saphenous veins to avoid confusion when abbreviations are used.[4] The saphenous veins are situated in a narrow anatomic space inside the superficial compartment, denominated the saphenous compartment (*compartimentum saphenum*). The saphenous compartment is bordered superficially by the saphenous fascia and deeply by the muscular fascia, and it contains the saphenous vein accompanied by the saphenous nerve. As a general rule, the accessory saphenous veins (*venae saphena accessoriae*) are situated outside this compartment, close to the dermis; however, the anterior accessory of the great saphenous vein at the proximal thigh courses deeply in the superficial compartment anteriorly to the great saphenous vein.[4,5] The structure of the superficial venous system of the lower extremity is presented in ► Fig. 1.4 and ► Fig. 1.5, with the nomenclature summarized in ► Table 1.2.

The veins of the dermis are arranged into two principal horizontal plexuses: the subpapillary venous plexus (*plexus venosus subpapillaris*) and the reticular venous plexus or deep dermal venous plexus (*plexus venosus dermalis profundus*). The subcutaneous tissue contains the subcutaneous venous plexus (*plexus venosus subcutaneus*), which drains into the superficial veins: the saphenous veins and their accessories, collaterals, and tributaries.[20,21]

1.4.1 The Great Saphenous Vein (*Vena Saphena Magna*)

The great saphenous vein (*vena saphena magna*), abbreviated as GSV, is the longest vein in the human body, starting at the medial side of the foot and draining into the common femoral vein at inguinal region, through the saphenofemoral junction. It passes anterior to the medial malleolus together with the saphenous nerve and ascends on the medial side of the leg. At the level of the knee, the great saphenous vein courses more posteriorly on the medial aspect of the joint away from the saphenous nerve, which is situated deeper in the thigh. The great saphenous vein then continues to travel alone on the medial side of the thigh, in the superficial compartment, crosses through the saphenous opening (former *fossa ovalis*), and terminates into the common femoral vein (*vena femoralis communis*) in the femoral canal (► Fig. 1.4, ► Fig. 1.5). The average diameter of a normal great saphenous vein is 3 to 4 mm, and the vessel features from 10 to 20 valves.[20] The great saphenous vein receives multiple tributaries along its course, and most of these vessels are located superficially outside the saphenous compartment. A variable number of perforator veins connect the GSV to the femoral (*vena femoralis*), posterior tibial (*venae tibiales posteriores*), gastrocnemius (*venae gastrocnemii*), and soleal veins (*venae soleales*) in the deep venous system.

The term confluence of superficial inguinal veins (*confluens venosus subinguinalis*) corresponds to the veins of the saphenofemoral junction (*junction saphenofemoralis*) and is applied to the most proximal segment of the great saphenous vein, close to the common femoral (► Fig. 1.6). These veins are located between the terminal valve (*valvula terminalis*), which is the last valve of the GSV, and preterminal valve (*valvula preterminalis*), which is situated 3 to 5 cm distally in the superior aspect of the thigh. From the anatomic concept, the saphenofemoral junction corresponds only to the saphenous opening into the femoral vein with the terminal valve. However, in a broader functional concept, the saphenofemoral junction is bounded proximally by the suprasaphenic valve in the common femoral vein and distally by the preterminal valve in the great saphenous vein, and by the infrasaphenic valve in the common femoral vein. This anatomic–functional concept also includes the terminations of the following tributaries that join the saphenofemoral junction: the superficial epigastric vein (*vena epigastrica superficialis*); the superficial circumflex iliac vein (*vena circumflexailium superficialis*); the superficial external pudendal vein (*vena pudenda externa superficialis*); the anterior and posterior accessory saphenous veins (*venae saphena magna accessoria anterior et posterior*); and the anterior and posterior thigh circumflex veins (*vena circumflexa femoris anterior et posterior*). The saphenofemoral junction may be correctly abbreviated as SFJ.[4,5,20,22,23]

A variable number of collateral veins of different lengths and diameters often accompany the great saphenous vein. The anatomic relationship between the GSV and these collaterals such as the anterior and posterior accessory great saphenous

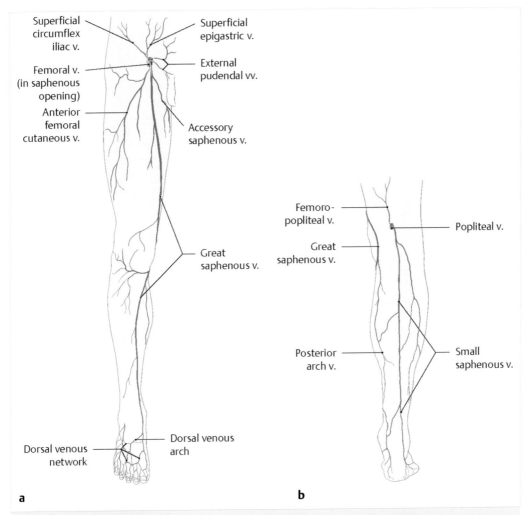

Fig. 1.4 The superficial venous system. (Reproduced with permission from Gilroy AM, MacPherson BR, Ross LM, Schuenke M, Schulte E, Schumacher U. Atlas of Anatomy. 2nd ed. New York, NY: Thieme; 2012. Illustration by Karl Wesker and Marcus Voll.)

veins (*venae saphena magna accessoria anterior et posterior*) and the superficial accessory great saphenous vein (*vena saphena magna accessoria superficialis*) is also variable and can be differentiated into three distinct anatomic patterns: in Type I, the great saphenous vein appears to be located in the saphenous compartment in its entirety, from the saphenofemoral junction to the distal lower extremity, and there are no major parallel collaterals; in Type H, the great saphenous vein extends through the length of the lower extremity, while there is a large collateral that is parallel to the GSV, located outside the saphenous compartment; in Type S, the great saphenous vein leaves the saphenous compartment at some level of the

lower extremity, continues distally as a superficial collateral, and is hypoplastic or absent in the distal segments of the saphenous compartment.[24,25]

The term anterior accessory great saphenous vein (*vena saphena magna accessoria anterior*) indicates any collateral venous segment situated anteriorly to the great saphenous vein both in the thigh and in the leg. The anterior accessory great saphenous vein ascends parallel and superficial to the GSV, frequently outside of the saphenous compartment. This accessory vein can approach the GSV and enter the saphenous compartment at the upper thigh. One or more anterior accessory great saphenous veins can be present with an average diameter of 2 to 5 mm.[4,5,20,26]

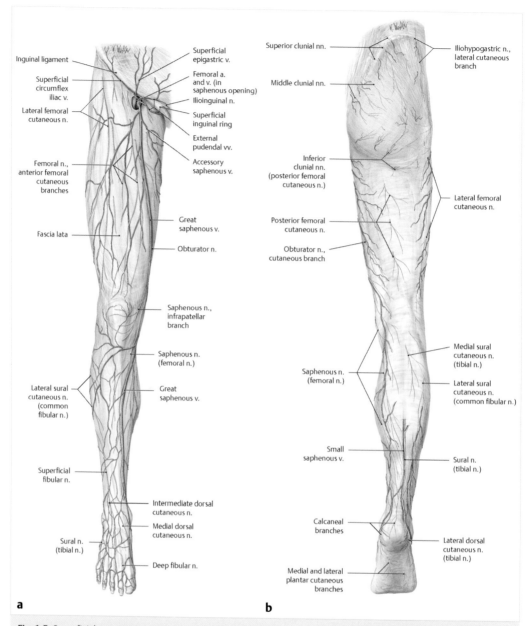

Fig. 1.5 Superficial cutaneous veins and nerves of the right lower limb. (Reproduced with permission from Gilroy AM, MacPherson BR, Ross LM, Schuenke M, Schulte E, Schumacher U. Atlas of Anatomy. 2nd ed. New York, NY: Thieme; 2012. Illustration by Karl Wesker and Marcus Voll.)

Similarly, the term posterior accessory great saphenous vein (*vena saphena magna accessoria posterior*) indicates any collateral venous segment that is situated posteriorly and medial to the great saphenous vein, either in the thigh or in the leg. This accessory vein usually does not enter the saphenous compartment.[4,5,20,26] The posterior accessory great saphenous vein of the leg, which starts behind the medial malleolus and then drains into the distal great saphenous vein, below the popliteal fossa, frequently communicates with perforator veins that connect with the posterior tibial veins.[21]

Table 1.2 Superficial veins of the lower extremity

Nomenclature	Official Latin term
Great saphenous vein	Vena saphena magna
Superficial epigastric vein	Vena epigastrica superficialis
Superficial circumflex iliac vein	Vena circumflexa ilium superficialis
Superficial external pudendal vein	Vena pudenda externa superficialis
Anterior accessory saphenous vein	Venae saphena magna accessoria anterior
Posterior accessory saphenous vein	Venae saphena magna accessoria posterior
Superficial accessory saphenous vein	Vena saphena magna accessoria superficialis
Anterior thigh circumflex vein	Vena circumflexa femoris anterior
Posterior thigh circumflex vein	Vena circumflexa femoris posterior
Small saphenous vein	Vena saphena parva
Cranial extension of the small saphenous vein	Extensio cranialis vena saphena parva
Giacomini vein	Vena Giacomini
Superficial accessory small saphenous vein	Vena saphena parva accessoria superficialis
Lateral venous system	Systema venosa lateralis membri inferioris

The superficial accessory great saphenous vein (*vena saphena magna accessoria superficialis*) is situated parallel to the GSV in a more superficial plane, above the saphenous fascia outside the saphenous compartment, both in the leg and in the thigh.[4,5]

The anterior thigh circumflex vein (*vena circumflexa femoris anterior*) is a tributary of the GSV or the anterior accessory great saphenous vein that ascends obliquely across the anterior thigh and may originate from the lateral venous system.[4,5]

The posterior thigh circumflex vein (*vena circumflexa femoris posterior*) is a tributary of the GSV or the posterior accessory great saphenous vein that ascends obliquely in the posterior thigh and collects blood from its posterior and medial aspects. The posterior thigh circumflex vein may originate from the lateral venous system or from a cranial extension of the small saphenous vein.[4,5]

1.4.2 The Small Saphenous Vein (*Vena Saphena Parva*)

The small saphenous vein (*vena saphena parva*) is the most important superficial vein of the leg and the second largest superficial vein of the lower extremity (▶ Fig. 1.4, ▶ Fig. 1.5). The small saphenous vein, correctly abbreviated as SSV, begins at the lateral aspect of the foot as the lateral marginal vein (*vena marginalis lateralis*) and ascends posterior to the lateral malleolus on the posterior aspect of the lower leg, together in proximity with the sural nerve, to the level of the apex of the calf. The SSV continues in the upper calf with the medial sural cutaneous nerve and crosses the deep fascia between the heads of the gastrocnemius muscle as it enters the popliteal fossa. The termination of the small saphenous vein is variable; however, in most cases, the vessel drains into the popliteal vein (*vena poplitea*) within 5 cm of the knee joint. Less frequently, the small saphenous vein terminates above the level of the popliteal fossa, either communicating with the great saphenous vein or draining directly into the deep venous system through a perforator vein. In a few cases, the small saphenous vein terminates below the level of the knee joint into the popliteal or gastrocnemius veins. The small saphenous vein usually measures 3 mm in diameter and contains from 7 to 13 valves. The SSV is accompanied by the small saphenous artery and may sporadically appear duplicated. It may also receive tributaries from the medial aspect of the ankle and communicate with medial ankle perforators.[20,27,28,29,30]

The saphenopopliteal junction (*junction saphenopoplitea*) corresponds to the terminal segment of the small saphenous vein between the terminal and the preterminal valves, and the segment of the popliteal vein between the suprasaphenic and the infrasaphenic valves. The estuary of the small saphenous vein into the popliteal vein is usually situated in the upper lateral quadrant of the popliteal fossa (▶ Fig. 1.7). However, there is significant variation in the small saphenous vein termination: the SSV joins the popliteal vein directly or via the gastrocnemius vein in the popliteal fossa in 50 to 80% of cases; terminates above the popliteal fossa in 15 to 47% of cases; or terminates distal to the popliteal fossa into the gastrocnemius or great saphenous veins in the posterior proximal calf in up to 10% of cases. Independently of the small saphenous vein termination, a large tributary or the SSV itself may extend cranially into the posterior thigh.[30,31,32,33,34,35]

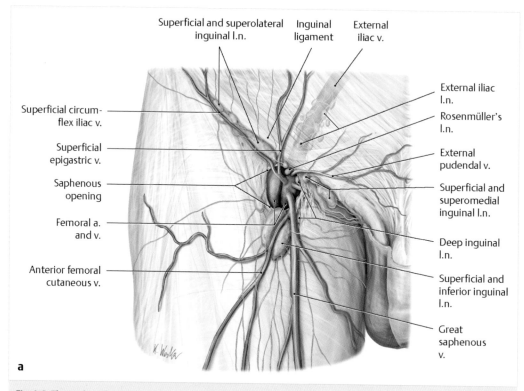

Fig. 1.6 The saphenofemoral junction. (*continued*) (a—reproduced with permission from Gilroy AM, MacPherson BR, Ross LM, Schuenke M, Schulte E, Schumacher U. Atlas of Anatomy. 2nd ed. New York, NY: Thieme; 2012. Illustration by Karl Wesker. b—reproduced with permission from Platzer W. Color of Human Anatomy, Volume 1: Locomotor System. Stuttgart: Thieme; 2013. Illustration by Gerhard Spitzer.)

The cranial extension of the small saphenous vein (*extensio cranialis vena saphena parva*) is the proximal continuation of the SSV in the posterior aspect of the thigh in the groove between the biceps femoris and semimembranosus muscles. The course of this vessel is variable in the proximal thigh as the cranial extension of the small saphenous vein can reach the gluteal region and communicate with gluteal veins (*venae gluteae*); continue as a perforator vein in the posterior thigh (*vena perforans femoris posterior*) draining into the profunda femoris vein (*vena profunda femoris*); or communicate with the great saphenous vein (*vena saphena magna*) through the Giacomini vein (*vena Giacomini*).[4,20]

The Giacomini vein (*vena Giacomini*) was first described in 1873 as a separate branch from the cranial continuation of the small saphenous vein (*vena saphena parva*) that communicates with the great saphenous vein (*vena saphena magna*), which was present in 44 of 51 (86.3%) limbs

studied by Giacomini.[36] The use of eponyms is discouraged; however, the term "Giacomini vein" is accepted to designate the medial thigh anastomosis between the small saphenous vein (*vena saphena parva*) and the great saphenous vein (*vena saphena magna*) or the posterior accessory great saphenous vein (*vena saphena magna accessoria posterior*).[5,20] Anatomically, the Giacomini vein is a posterior thigh circumflex vein (*vena circumflexa femoris posterior*), a communicating vein of the superficial system that is smaller in diameter in comparison with the GSV and may be associated with perforator veins in the thigh.[20,31]

The superficial accessory small saphenous vein (*vena saphena parva accessoria superficialis*) ascends parallel to the small saphenous vein (*vena saphena parva*) in the posterior aspect of the leg but is located in a more superficial plane above the saphenous compartment. This accessory vein drains into the proximal segment of the SSV.[4,5,20]

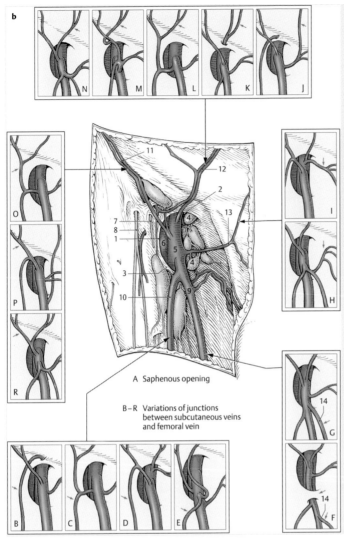

Fig. 1.6 (*continued*) The saphenofemoral junction. (a—reproduced with permission from Gilroy AM, MacPherson BR, Ross LM, Schuenke M, Schulte E, Schumacher U. Atlas of Anatomy. 2nd ed. New York, NY: Thieme; 2012. Illustration by Karl Wesker. b—reproduced with permission from Platzer W. Color of Human Anatomy, Volume 1: Locomotor System. Stuttgart: Thieme; 2013. Illustration by Gerhard Spitzer.)

A Saphenous opening

B–R Variations of junctions between subcutaneous veins and femoral vein

1.4.3 The Lateral Venous System

The lateral venous system (*systema venosa lateralis membri inferioris*) extends on the lateral aspect of the thigh and leg and represents a development remnant of the embryonic lateral marginal vein (*vena marginalis lateralis*). During the development of the lower extremity venous system, the embryonic lateral marginal vein (*vena marginalis lateralis*) regresses and is replaced by the great saphenous and small saphenous veins and their collaterals and tributaries. However, the lateral venous system may persist as plexus of subcutaneous veins in the lateral aspect of the inferior limb that fails to involute, and drains from the thigh and the leg toward the region of the knee. The lateral venous system (*systema venosa lateralis membri inferioris*) then communicates with the deep venous system through perforator veins. The lateral venous system can also communicate with the great saphenous vein (*vena saphena magna*) through the anterior thigh circumflex vein (*vena circumflexa femoris anterior*).[4,5,20,37]

1.5 Perforating Veins

By definition, the perforating veins or perforators cross the deep muscular fascia that separates the superficial and deep compartments, and connect the superficial venous system to the deep venous system. The perforating veins are numerous and variable in arrangement, size, and distribution.

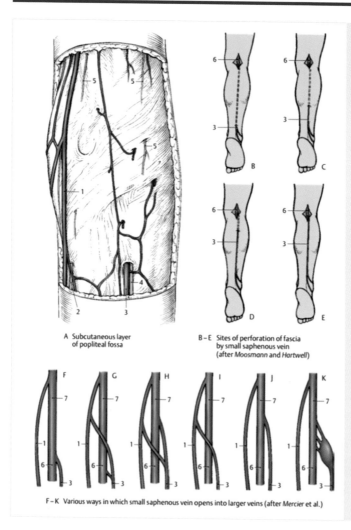

Fig. 1.7 The saphenopopliteal junction. (Reproduced with permission from Platzer W. Color of Human Anatomy, Volume 1: Locomotor System. Stuttgart: Thieme; 2013. Illustration by Gerhard Spitzer.)

A Subcutaneous layer of popliteal fossa

B–E Sites of perforation of fascia by small saphenous vein (after *Moosmann* and *Hartwell*)

F–K Various ways in which small saphenous vein opens into larger veins (after *Mercier* et al.)

These vessels originate from the superficial venous system and join the main vessels of the deep venous system, either directly or indirectly through connections with smaller veins in the muscles. The valves featured in the perforating veins allow the blood flow from the superficial to the deep veins.[4,38,39] The perforating veins are grouped on the basis of their topography, as demonstrated in ▶ Table 1.3 and ▶ Fig. 1.8.

The perforating veins of the foot (*venae perforantes pedis*) are divided into four different groups, depending on the location of the vessels: the dorsal foot perforators or intercapitular veins; the medial foot perforators; the lateral foot perforators; and the plantar foot perforators.[4,40]

The perforating veins of the ankle (*venae perforantes tarsalis*) are divided into three different groups according to their topography: the medial ankle perforators; the anterior ankle perforators; and the lateral ankle perforators.[4,40]

The perforating veins of the leg (*venae perforantes cruris*) are divided into four main groups according to their topography: the anterior leg perforators; the medial leg perforators; the lateral leg perforators; and the posterior leg perforators.[4,40] The most important perforating veins of the lower extremity are the medial leg perforators, which are divided into two groups: the paratibial perforators and the posterior tibial perforators.[4,39] The paratibial perforators connect the main trunk or tributaries of the great saphenous vein (*vena saphena magna*) with the posterior tibial veins (*venae tibiales posteriores*), and course close to the medial surface of the tibia.[4] The posterior tibial perforators, also referred to as the Cockett's perforators, connect the posterior accessory great

Table 1.3 Perforating veins of the lower extremity

Nomenclature	Official Latin Term
Perforating veins of the foot	*Venae perforantes pedis*
Dorsal foot perforators	
Medial foot perforators	
Lateral foot perforators	
Plantar foot perforators	
Perforating veins of the ankle	*Venae perforantes tarsalis*
Medial ankle perforators	
Anterior ankle perforators	
Lateral ankle perforators	
Perforating veins of the leg	*Venae perforantes cruris*
Anterior leg perforators	
Medial leg perforators	
Lateral leg perforators	
Posterior leg perforators	
Perforating veins of the knee	*Venae perforantes genus*
Suprapatellar perforators	
Infrapatellar perforators	
Medial knee perforators	
Lateral knee perforators	
Popliteal fossa perforators	
Perforating veins of the thigh	*Venae perforantes femoris*
Anterior thigh perforators	
Medial thigh perforators	
Lateral thigh perforators	
Posterior thigh perforators	
Perforating veins of the gluteal muscles	*Venae perforantes glutealis*
Superior gluteal perforators	
Midgluteal perforators	
Lower gluteal perforators	

saphenous vein (*vena saphena magna accessoria posterior*) with the posterior tibial veins (*venae tibiales posteriores*) and should be subdivided topographically into upper, middle, and lower perforators.[21,41] The anterior leg perforators connect the anterior tributaries of the great saphenous vein (*vena saphena magna*) with the anterior tibial veins (*venae tibiales anteriores*).[4] The lateral leg perforators connect the veins of the lateral venous system (*systema venosa lateralis membri inferioris*) with the fibular veins (*venae fibulares*).[4,37] The posterior leg perforators are divided into four groups: the medial gastrocnemius perforators; the lateral gastrocnemius perforators; the intergemellar perforators; and the para-Achillean perforators.[4]

The perforating veins of the knee (*venae perforantes genus*) are divided into five different groups according to their topography: the suprapatellar perforators; the infrapatellar perforators; the medial knee perforators; the lateral knee perforators; and the popliteal fossa perforators.[4]

The perforating veins of the thigh (*venae perforantes femoris*) are divided into four different groups according to their topography: the anterior thigh perforators; the medial thigh perforators; the lateral thigh perforators; and the posterior thigh perforators. The medial thigh perforators include the perforators of the femoral canal and the inguinal perforators, which connect the main trunk or tributaries of the great saphenous vein (*vena saphena magna*) with the femoral vein (*vena femoralis*).[4] The posterior thigh perforators include the posteromedial thigh perforators, the sciatic perforators, the posterolateral thigh perforators, and the pudendal perforators.[4]

The perforating veins of the gluteal muscles (*venae perforantes glutealis*) are divided into three different groups according to their topography: the superior gluteal perforators; the midgluteal perforators; and the lower gluteal perforators.[4]

1.6 General Terminology

Different techniques and imaging modalities such as postmortem[34,36] and operative dissections,[41] venography,[35] ultrasound examination, and more recently three-dimensional computed tomography[42] and magnetic resonance imaging venography[43] have been used to investigate the lower extremity venous system.

Normal diameters of the veins of the lower extremity can show a great variability, and developmental abnormalities may also cause segmental

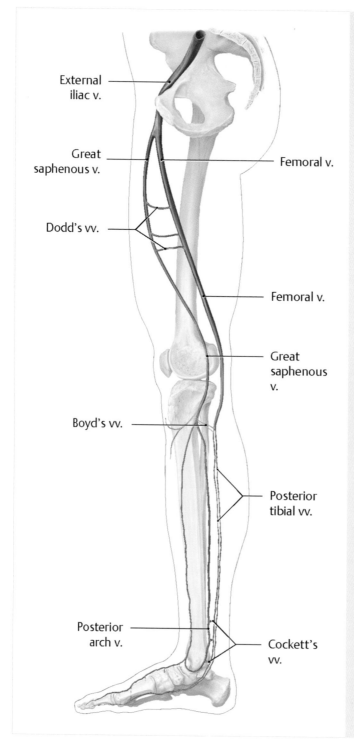

External
iliac v.

Great
saphenous v.

Dodd's vv.

Boyd's vv.

Posterior
arch v.

Femoral v.

Femoral v.

Great
saphenous
v.

Posterior
tibial vv.

Cockett's
vv.

Fig. 1.8 The perforating veins. (Reproduced with permission from Gilroy AM, MacPherson BR, Ross LM, Schuenke M, Schulte E, Schumacher U. Atlas of Anatomy. 2nd ed. New York, NY: Thieme; 2012. Illustration by Karl Wesker and Marcus Voll.)

differences in the size of the vein. The terminology recommended in a consensus document developed in 2004[5] is presented:

- *Agenesis*: It indicates the complete absence of a vein or of a segment of a vein.
- *Aplasia*: It indicates the lack of development of a vein or of a segment of a vein. The vein is present but diminutive in size, and its structure is similar to that in the embryo.
- *Hypoplasia*: It indicates the incomplete development of a vein or of a segment of a vein. It is less severe in degree than aplasia, and the hypoplastic vein has a reduced caliber with a normal structure.
- *Dysplasia*: It indicates a complex abnormality of development of a vein or of a group of veins that greatly differs from the normal conditions in size, structure, and connections.
- *Atrophy*: It indicates a decrease in size or wasting away of a normally developed vein or segment of a vein, following a degenerative process. Wall changes are different, according to the nature of the degenerative process.
- *Venous aneurysm*: It indicates a localized dilation of a venous segment, with a caliber increase > 50% compared with normal.
- *Venomegalia*: It designates diffuse dilation of one or more veins with a caliber increase > 50% compared with normal.

This consensus document[5] also recommends that the adjectives "proximal" and "distal," when referred to venous structures, should be used in the following manner: "proximal" is toward the heart, and "distal" is away from the heart. The use of the term "double" is recommended when two veins show the same path, topography, and relationships.

References

[1] Federative International Committee for Anatomical Terminology. Terminologia Anatomica. Stuttgart: George Thieme Verlag; 1998

[2] Bundens WP, Bergan JJ, Halasz NA, Murray J, Drehobl M. The superficial femoral vein. A potentially lethal misnomer. JAMA. 1995; 274(16):1296–1298

[3] Bergan JJ. Editor's note. Venous Digest 1999;6:5

[4] Caggiati A, Bergan JJ, Gloviczki P, Jantet G, Wendell-Smith CP, Partsch H, International Interdisciplinary Consensus Committee on Venous Anatomical Terminology. Nomenclature of the veins of the lower limbs: an international interdisciplinary consensus statement. J Vasc Surg. 2002; 36(2):416–422

[5] Caggiati A, Bergan JJ, Gloviczki P, Eklof B, Allegra C, Partsch H, International Interdisciplinary Consensus Committee on Venous Anatomical Terminology. Nomenclature of the veins

[6] Braverman IM. The cutaneous microcirculation: ultrastructure and microanatomical organization. Microcirculation. 1997; 4(3):329–340

[7] Wokalek H, Vanscheidt W, Martay K, Leder O. Morphology and localization of sunburst varicosities: an electron microscopic and morphometric study. J Dermatol Surg Oncol. 1989; 15(2):149–154

[8] Leu HJ, Vogt M, Pfrunder H. Morphological alterations of non-varicose and varicose veins. (A morphological contribution to the discussion on pathogenesis of varicose veins). Basic Res Cardiol. 1979; 74(4):435–444

[9] Edwards JE, Edwards AE. The saphenous valves in varicose veins. Am Heart J. 1940; 19(3):338–351

[10] Popoff N. The digital vascular system. Arch Pathol (Chic). 1934; 18:307–322

[11] Caggiati A, Phillips M, Lametschwandtner A, Allegra C. Valves in small veins and venules. Eur J Vasc Endovasc Surg. 2006; 32(4):447–452

[12] Coghlan D. Overview of anatomy of the deep and superficial venous system of the lower leg. ASUM Ultrasound Bull. 2005; 8:28–33

[13] Kachlik D, Pechacek V, Musil V, Baca V. The deep venous system of the lower extremity: new nomenclature. Phlebology. 2012; 27(2):48–58

[14] Dona E, Fletcher JP, Hughes TM, Saker K, Batiste P, Ramanathan I. Duplicated popliteal and superficial femoral veins: incidence and potential significance. Aust N Z J Surg. 2000; 70(6):438–440

[15] Gottlob R, May R. Venous Valves: Morphology, Function, Radiology, Surgery. New York, NY: Springer; 1986

[16] Aragão JA, Reis FP, Pitta GB, Miranda F, Jr, Poli de Figueiredo LF. Anatomical study of the gastrocnemius venous network and proposal for a classification of the veins. Eur J Vasc Endovasc Surg. 2006; 31(4):439–442

[17] Gordon AC, Wright I, Pugh ND. Duplication of the superficial femoral vein: recognition with duplex ultrasonography. Clin Radiol. 1996; 51(9):622–624

[18] Uhl JF, Gillot C, Chahim M. Anatomical variations of the femoral vein. J Vasc Surg. 2010; 52(3):714–719

[19] Cherry KJ, Gloviczki P, Stanson AW. Persistent sciatic vein: diagnosis and treatment of a rare condition. J Vasc Surg. 1996; 23(3):490–497

[20] Kachlik D, Pechacek V, Baca V, Musil V. The superficial venous system of the lower extremity: new nomenclature. Phlebology. 2010; 25(3):113–123

[21] Mozes G, Gloviczki P. New discoveries in anatomy and new terminology of leg veins: clinical implications. Vasc Endovascular Surg. 2004; 38(4):367–374

[22] Staubesand J, Steel F, Li Y. The official nomenclature of the superficial veins of the lower limb: a case for revision. Clin Anat. 1995; 8(6):426–428

[23] Meissner MH. Lower extremity venous anatomy. Semin Intervent Radiol. 2005; 22(3):147–156

[24] Ricci S, Georgiev M. Ultrasound anatomy of the superficial veins of the lower limb. J Vasc Technol. 2002; 26:183–199

[25] Ricci S, Caggiati A. Echoanatomical patterns of the long saphenous vein in patients with primary varices and in healthy subjects. Phlebology. 1999; 14:54–58

[26] Cohn JD, Caggiati A, Korver KF. Accessory and great saphenous veins as coronary artery bypass conduits. Interact Cardiovasc Thorac Surg. 2006; 5(5):550–554

[27] O'Donnell TF, Jr, Iafrati MD. The small saphenous vein and other 'neglected' veins of the popliteal fossa: a review. Phlebology. 2007; 22(4):148–155

[28] Caggiati A. Fascial relationships of the short saphenous vein. J Vasc Surg. 2001; 34(2):241–246

[29] Schadeck M. Sclerotherapy of small saphenous vein: how to avoid bad results. Phlebologie. 2004; 57:165–169

[30] Uhl JF, Gillot C. Anatomy and embryology of the small saphenous vein: nerve relationships and implications for treatment. Phlebology. 2013; 28(1):4–15

[31] Delis KT, Knaggs AL, Khodabakhsh P. Prevalence, anatomic patterns, valvular competence, and clinical significance of the Giacomini vein. J Vasc Surg. 2004; 40(6):1174–1183

[32] Balasubramaniam R, Rai R, Berridge DC, Scott DJ, Soames RW. The relationship between the saphenopopliteal junction and the common peroneal nerve: a cada-veric study. Phlebology. 2009; 24(2):67–73

[33] Pittathankal AA, Adamson M, Pursell R, Richards T, Galland RB, Magee TR. Duplex-defined spatial anatomy of the saphenopopliteal junction. Phlebology. 2006; 21:45–47

[34] Kosinski C. Observations on the superficial venous system of the lower extremity. J Anat. 1926; 60(Pt 2):131–142

[35] Lea Thomas M, Chan O. Anatomical variations of the short saphenous vein: a phlebographic study. Vasa. 1988; 17(1):51–55

[36] Giacomini C. Osservazioni anatomiche per servire allo studio della circolazione venosa delle estremita inferiori. Parte I: Delle vene superficiali dell'arto addominale e principalmente della saphena esterna. G R Accad Med Torino. 1873; 14:109–136

[37] Albanese AR, Albanese AM, Albanese EF. Lateral subdermic varicose vein system of the legs. Its surgical treatment by the chiseling tube method. Vasc Surg. 1969; 3(2):81–89

[38] Mozes G, Kadar A, Carmichael SW. Surgical anatomy of the perforating veins. In: Gloviczki P, ed. Atlas of Endoscopic Perforator Vein Surgery. London: Springer-Verlag; 1998:17–28

[39] Meissner MH, Moneta G, Burnand K, et al. The hemodynamics and diagnosis of venous disease. J Vasc Surg. 2007; 46 Suppl S:4S–24S

[40] Kuster G, Lofgren EP, Hollinshead WH. Anatomy of the veins of the foot. Surg Gynecol Obstet. 1968; 127(4):817–823

[41] Dodd H, Cockett FB. The Pathology and Surgery of the Veins of the Lower Limb. 2nd ed. Edinburgh: Churchill Livingstone; 1976

[42] Lee W, Chung JW, Yin YH, et al. Three-dimensional CT venography of varicose veins of the lower extremity: image quality and comparison with doppler sonography. AJR Am J Roentgenol. 2008; 191(4):1186–1191

[43] Müller MA, Mayer D, Seifert B, Marincek B, Willmann JK. Recurrent lower-limb varicose veins: effect of direct contrast-enhanced three-dimensional MR venographic findings on diagnostic thinking and therapeutic decisions. Radiology. 2008; 247(3):887–895

2 Pathophysiology of Varicose Veins

Amy R. Deipolyi and Gloria M. Martinez Salazar

2.1 Introduction

Chronic venous disorders (CVDs) refer to a wide range of venous disease entities, including mild conditions such as varicose veins and telangiectasias and more severe presentations such as edema and venous ulceration.[1] Most patients with CVD have a primary disease of the vein wall with resultant valvular dysfunction in the superficial veins, leading to venous reflux.[1] Chronic venous insufficiency (CVI) refers more specifically to a progressive syndrome including symptoms and signs, such as discomfort and skin changes, due to sustained venous hypertension.[2] CVI is common, initially presenting as symptomatic venous varicosities that can progress to more severe conditions.

The prevalence of CVI in the western world varies from 1 to 40% in females and from 1 to 17% in males, and is higher in industrialized nations.[3] Reported estimated prevalence of varicose veins ranges from 1 to 73% in females and 2 to 56% in males.[4] Risk factors include prolonged standing or sitting, hormonal influences, pregnancy, female gender, and advanced age.[3,5] In addition to cosmetic complaints, most people with varicose veins do experience symptoms such as lower extremity heaviness, pain, swelling, eczema, pigmentation, hemorrhage, and ulceration.[6]

Despite the commonness of CVI, its pathogenesis is poorly understood, and may vary among individuals with similar presenting features. The first step in evaluating patients with symptoms suspicious for CVI is to identify the anatomic level of the disease, and then determine the patterns of venous reflux to guide appropriate therapy. Success of potential treatments depends on the understanding of the pathogenesis of varicose veins, which in turn is based on the understanding of venous anatomy. This chapter reviews the relevant anatomy of the superficial and deep venous system of the lower extremity, correlating with the current understanding of the anatomic and pathophysiologic causes of varicose veins.

2.2 Histology of the Lower Extremity Venous System

Veins are thin-walled vessels that return deoxygenated blood to the heart and collapse when empty. The innermost layer of the vein wall is the tunica intima, which is a lining of endothelial cells. The middle layer is the tunica media, consisting of bands of smooth muscle; this layer is thin in comparison with arteries of the same diameter. The thick outermost layer, the tunica adventitia or tunica externa, is composed of connective tissue (Chapter 1, ▶ Fig. 1.2). Compared with the arterial system, there is substantial anatomic variation in the location and branching pattern of veins.[7]

Normal venous histology demonstrates valves in both superficial and deep leg veins, which permit unidirectional blood flow against the force of gravity back toward the heart.[8] Normal vein walls contain bundles of collagen fibers that prevent overdistention and organized elastin fibers that provide elastic recoil.[9]

2.3 Physiology of the Lower Extremity Venous System

Lower extremity venous pressure is determined by the following: (1) the inflow of blood regulated by arterial mechanisms; (2) the ability of the calf muscle and venous valves to return blood to the heart; and (3) the absence of upstream venous obstruction. When these mechanisms fail, lower extremity venous hypertension and ultimately CVI ensue (▶ Fig. 2.1).[10,11]

2.3.1 Muscular Venous Pump

The main mechanism to promote venous return occurs in the deep venous system through the action of three muscular pumps: the foot, calf, and thigh. Venous return is accomplished primarily by the pumping mechanism of the calf, with an ejection fraction of 65%, compared to an ejection fraction of 15% in the thigh.[10] The calf muscular pump generates roughly 200 mm Hg when contracting, while venous valves prevent backflow of blood.[11] Accordingly, due to the calf muscular pump, pressures ranging from 20 to 100 mm Hg are accommodated.[11] Reduction in the deep venous pressure during the postcontraction relaxation phase promotes flow from the superficial to the deep system via the perforating veins.

One study showed that deficiencies in the calf muscular pump correlate with severity of venous

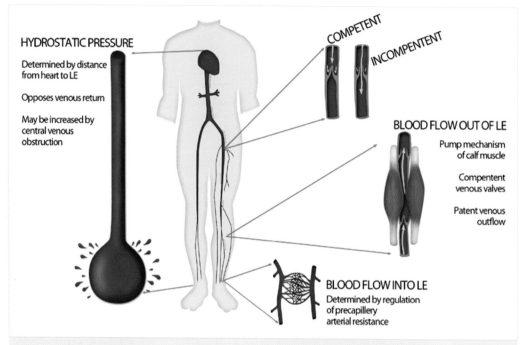

HYDROSTATIC PRESSURE

Determined by distance from heart to LE

Opposes venous return

May be increased by central venous obstruction

COMPETENT

INCOMPETENT

BLOOD FLOW OUT OF LE

Pump mechanism of calf muscle

Compentent venous valves

Patent venous outflow

BLOOD FLOW INTO LE

Determined by regulation of precapillery arterial resistance

Fig. 2.1 Schematic demonstration of determinants of lower extremity (LE) venous pressure. LE venous pressure is determined by the inflow and outflow of blood in the lower extremity, and by the hydrostatic pressure of the column of venous blood returning to the heart.

ulceration,[12] though another study indicated that clinical severity of CVI correlated with venous reflux and not calf ejection fraction.[13] Therefore, while the muscle pump of the calf is key in returning blood to the heart from the lower extremity, it is not entirely clear whether deficiencies in pump action play a primary etiologic role in CVI.

2.3.2 Functional Anatomy of the Lower Extremity Venous System

Understanding the etiology of venous disease requires a thorough understanding of normal venous anatomy. Disease can be localized as either superficial or deep to the muscular fascia. The superficial and deep systems are interconnected through the perforating veins. Proper functional antegrade flow of blood through these vessels is ensured by competent bicuspid valves, associated with an effective muscular pumping mechanism. The valves divide the hydrostatic column of blood into segments, and establish flow from superficial to deep and from caudal to cephalic.[10] For more information and detail on the anatomy of the lower extremity venous system, please refer to Chapter 1.

Deep Venous System

Approximately 90% of the venous return in the lower extremities occurs through the deep veins, via the muscular pump described earlier. The deep veins include iliac, femoral, popliteal, calf, perforators, and intramuscular veins. Calf deep veins, distinguished by valves every 3 to 5 cm, include the tibial and peroneal veins, as well as soleal and gastrocnemius muscular sinuses. The gastrocnemius veins enter the popliteal veins at the popliteal fossa (▶ Fig. 2.2).

The muscle veins of the calf can be considered as a separate group because of their function as calf muscle pump. The deep fascia of the leg invests all of the calf muscles very firmly and restrains outward bulging of the muscles during contraction. During relaxation, the pressure in the emptied deep veins is lower than in the superficial system and blood is drawn into the deep venous system via the perforating veins.[14]

The perforating veins are also part of the deep venous system (▶ Fig. 2.2). Clinically important perforating veins include the veins of Cockett connecting the posterior tibial veins with the posterior arch vein or the main stem of the great saphenous vein (GSV), and Dodd's veins which are

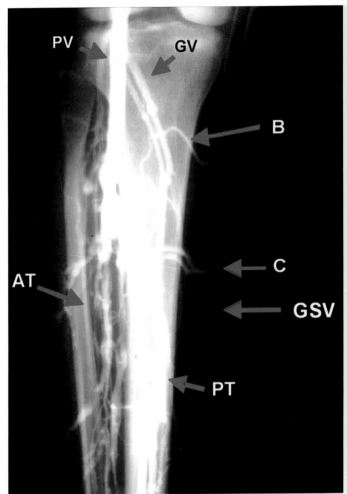

Fig. 2.2 Venogram of the distal right lower extremity demonstrating normal venous anatomy: popliteal vein (PV), gastrocnemius vein (GV), anterior tibial vein (AT), posterior tibial vein (PT), great saphenous vein (GSV), and Boyd's (B) and Cockett's (C) perforating veins. The perforating veins connect the superficial venous system to the deep venous system.

a group of three to five perforating veins from the GSV to the femoral vein (Chapter 1, ▶ Fig. 2.8). Isolated segmental reflux in the main trunks may raise the possibility of an incompetent perforating-mediated venous reflux mechanism. Diagnosis of incompetent perforating veins is important for treatment planning and clinical success of the intervention. Incompetent perforating veins may be classified by anatomic location and level.[15]

Superficial Venous System

The superficial venous system, located between the subcutaneous tissue and the deep fascia, has two main divisions: the GSV and the small saphenous vein (SSV) (Chapter 1, ▶ Fig. 1.4, ▶ Fig. 1.5). This system also includes the reticular veins that run parallel to the skin surface that drains the lower extremities' skin and subcutaneous tissue.[10,16] Reticular veins are important in the pathogenesis of telangiectasias, but are less important in the context of CVI.[10]

Anatomy of the Saphenofemoral Junction and GSV

The saphenofemoral junction (SFJ) is the junction of the GSV and common femoral vein (▶ Fig. 2.3). The GSV proximal valve is located 1 to 3 cm distal to its actual entry point into the common femoral vein. In normal patients, during intermittent Valsalva's maneuver, some blood may flow back toward the lower extremity, but never beyond the second valve. The main trunk of the GSV usually has at least six valves,[17] and lies in the subcutaneous tissue superficial to the muscular fascia in the saphenous compartment, which consists of a space outlined anteriorly by the saphenous fascia and posteriorly by the muscular fascia.[18]

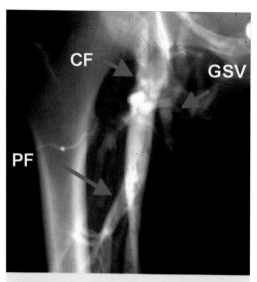

Fig. 2.3 Venogram of the proximal right lower extremity demonstrating normal venous anatomy: common femoral vein (CF), profunda femoris vein (PF), and great saphenous vein (GSV). Saphenofemoral junction: the GSV joins the common femoral vein (CF), 3 to 4 cm inferior and lateral to the pubic tubercle.

In the thigh and calf, the GSV runs along the anteromedial aspect of the lower extremity (▶ Fig. 2.2). In the calf, the tributaries of the GSV consist of two main trunks: the anterior branch and the posterior arch vein, which arises behind the medial malleolus and joins the GSV distal to the knee.[19] The two major tributaries in the thigh ascend parallel to the GSV—the anterior and posterior accessory saphenous veins—and are located external to the saphenous fascia.[20]

Anatomy of the Saphenopopliteal Junction and SSV

The saphenopopliteal junction is the junction of the SSV with the popliteal vein. The SSV usually enters the popliteal vein above the knee joint in a discrete loop from lateral to dorsal direction; however, there is significant variation in the termination of the SSV.[21]

The SSV drains the lateral aspect of the foot and heel, but several communicating veins pass medially to join the venous arches at the medial aspect of the ankle. The SSV usually has 7 to 10 spaced valves.[17] A cranial extension of the SSV (vein of Giacomini) ascends posteriorly in the thigh to communicate with the GSV through the posterior thigh circumflex vein.[20]

Identifying the Level of Venous Disease

There are several patterns of venous insufficiency (▶ Fig. 2.4, ▶ Fig. 2.5, ▶ Fig. 2.6). It is important to understand the pathophysiology of venous insufficiency as these different reflux patterns may require different therapeutic approaches. Incompetence at the SFJ with truncal reflux along the GSV is one of the patterns of reflux seen with incompetent GSV at its entire length or up to the level of the thigh, with dilation of all branches (▶ Fig. 2.4). The tributaries can be implicated in mechanisms of venous reflux at the GSV territory, with reflux seen at the SFJ and then into an anterior tributary or reflux in the anterior tributary and then joining the GSV (▶ Fig. 2.5). One important pattern of venous reflux is saphenofemoral incompetence and reflux into the posterior accessory GSV connecting with the SSV (▶ Fig. 2.6).

Factors Influencing Function of Lower Extremity Venous System

Accepted risk factors for CVI include family history, increasing age, pregnancy, female gender, obesity, and occupations demanding more constant orthostasis.[4] These risk factors suggest that hormonal status and posture significantly impact the function of the venous system. Circulating estradiol is frequently associated with primary CVI, suggesting the importance of hormonal influences on venous function.[22] While studies have shown that estradiol infusion increases venous volume in the calf, likely through venodilation,[23] other studies have yielded conflicting results.[24]

In addition to hormonal influences, temperature may also play a role in CVI. Elevated skin temperature is associated with increased risk of CVI, and particularly with more severe sequelae including ulceration.[25] Increased local temperature, possibly due to venous stasis, alters control of sympathetic function, leading to worsening of CVI.[26] Prolonged orthostasis results in pooling of blood in the lower extremities, with persistently elevated venous pressures, that can lead to venous wall and valvular damage. Persistently increased hematocrit levels due to blood pooling could also result in a prothrombotic state.[27]

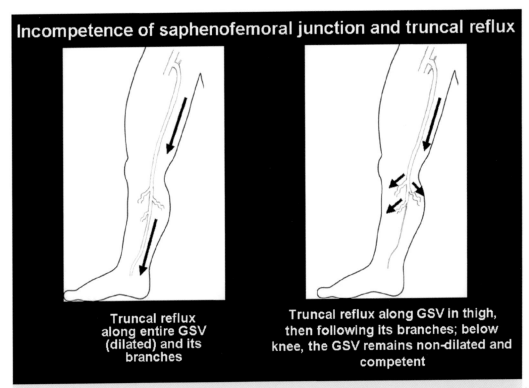

Fig. 2.4 Schematic illustration of different patterns of venous reflux in the great saphenous vein (GSV): incompetence of saphenofemoral junction and truncal reflux. **(a)** Truncal reflux along entire GSV (dilated) and its branches. **(b)** Truncal reflux along GSV in thigh, then following its branches; below knee, the GSV remains nondilated and competent.

2.4 Pathophysiology of Chronic Venous Insufficiency

CVI is thought to be caused by a constellation of factors, including alterations in the vein wall, valvular disorders, and deep venous hypertension. Primary valvular insufficiency, arising from intrinsic biochemical and structural changes, is most often associated with truncal saphenous insufficiency.[2] Secondary valvular insufficiency usually follows acute deep venous thrombosis (DVT). Whereas primary CVI is primarily due to reflux, secondary CVI is due to both a reflux and an upstream obstruction.[28]

2.4.1 Deep Venous Hypertension

Elevated deep venous pressure may be due to proximal/central or distal/peripheral causes. Proximal causes include pelvic masses resulting in venous outflow obstruction, obesity, constrictive clothing, prolonged sitting, or increased intra-abdominal pressure from straining during micturition or defecation.[9] Physiologic and clinical studies suggest that iliac vein obstruction is the most significant contributor to symptomatic venous outflow obstruction.[13] Obstructive lesions of the inferior vena cava (IVC) appear to produce less lower extremity outflow obstruction compared with iliac venous lesions, because of the greater opportunity for venous collateralization.[13] Nonthrombotic iliac venous obstruction occurs in as many as 60% of asymptomatic individuals, but are present in 90% of symptomatic individuals.[29] May–Thurner anatomy, the most common iliac venous obstructive lesion, is caused by extrinsic compression of the left common iliac vein between the overlying right common iliac artery and the underlying lumbar vertebra or sacrum (▶ Fig. 2.7). Other causes of upstream venous outflow obstruction secondary to extrinsic iliac venous or caval compression can include bone spurs or outgrowths, arterial aneurysms, benign and malignant pelvic/abdominal masses, inflammatory processes, and retroperitoneal fibrosis.

Peripheral causes of deep venous hypertension include arteriovenous anastomoses, incompetent

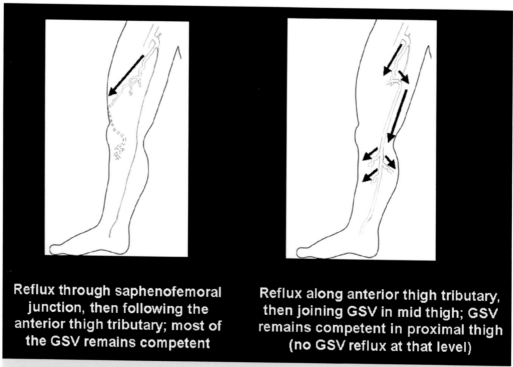

Reflux through saphenofemoral junction, then following the anterior thigh tributary; most of the GSV remains competent

Reflux along anterior thigh tributary, then joining GSV in mid thigh; GSV remains competent in proximal thigh (no GSV reflux at that level)

Fig. 2.5 Patterns of venous reflux involving the anterior accessory great saphenous vein. **(a)** Reflux through saphenofemoral junction, then following the anterior thigh tributary; most of the GSV remains competent. **(b)** Reflux along anterior thigh tributary, then joining GSV in midthigh; GSV remains competent in proximal thigh (no GSV reflux at that level).

perforator veins, and intraluminal venous obstructions.[9] Abnormal arteriovenous connections lead to increased venous pressure secondary to arterialization of the veins. Additionally, incompetent perforating veins are an important peripheral source of deep venous hypertension. They are typically found in the middle and lower portions of the calf, and their prevalence increases with increasing clinical severity of CVI. Incompetent perforating veins most frequently are found in association with deep venous incompetence.[15]

Elevated deep venous pressures will be transmitted to the superficial venous system in cases of valvular incompetence, which would allow backflow of venous blood from the deep to superficial system. Patients with deep venous disease may have a primary (idiopathic) or secondary (post-thrombotic) forms. Isolated reflux in a perforating vein or segmental deep venous reflux is generally asymptomatic with multilevel reflux required for symptomatic presentation.[29] Deep venous reflux is commonly observed in patients who fail conservative treatment, and correction of this component is associated with good clinical outcomes.[30]

2.4.2 Primary Valvular Incompetence

Primary venous disease occurs in the absence of an inciting episode of venous thrombosis. Currently, the pathogenesis of primary venous disease is poorly understood. Varicose veins are defined as tortuous, palpable, and dilated veins larger than 4 mm, typically associated with saphenous insufficiency (▶ Fig. 2.8). Varicose veins are characterized by decreased compliance and contractility and reduced smooth muscle content. Due to weakening of the vein wall, the vein dilates, stretching the valve cusp commissure and separating the leaflets.[10] Compared with normal veins, in CVI valve leaflets are stretched, torn, thinned, and adhered, with an overall reduction in the number of valves per unit length.[31] Abnormal valve leaflets are infiltrated with leukocytes.[32]

Reflux is the primary hemodynamic abnormality in primary venous disease, though varicose vein changes can precede valvular incompetence, suggesting that valvular dysfunction may be a secondary phenomenon.[10] More recent attention has

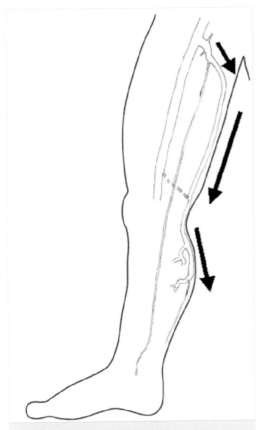

Fig. 2.6 Schematic representation of incompetent posterior accessory GSV and SSV reflux pattern. A cranial extension of the SSV, called the vein of Giacomini, ascends posteriorly in the thigh and communicates with the GSV or the posterior accessory GSV, representing an important pattern of venous reflux. There is saphenofemoral incompetence and venous reflux into the posterior thigh tributary connecting with the SSV.

emphasized structural abnormalities of the vein wall and the extracellular matrix (ECM). According to more modern theories, varicose veins may develop due to alterations in venous tone in combination with underlying connective tissue deficits.[33] Structural changes in the vein wall include hypertrophy and disrupted smooth muscle cell and elastin fiber arrangement.[31] In CVI, balanced collagen synthesis is disturbed, with increased collagen type I and decreased collagen type III, leading to vein wall weakness and reduced elasticity.[34]

Alterations of the ECM are also seen in CVI. ECM homeostasis is controlled by a host of proteolytic enzymes, such as serine proteinases and matrix metalloproteinases, which are secreted by inflammatory and vascular cells, but also inhibited by tissue inhibitors.[31] Alterations in this balance result in accumulation of ECM in varicose veins, further weakening the vein wall. Additionally, alterations of levels of proteolytic enzymes and cytokines likely underlie the variable hypertrophic and atrophic changes observed in CVI vein walls.[31]

2.4.3 Secondary Valvular Incompetence

Secondary venous insufficiency occurs after an episode of lower extremity DVT, and is due to a combination of reflux and obstruction. Despite recanalization over 6 to 12 months, chronic luminal changes and persistent partial obstruction lead to reflux and deep venous hypertension.[28] For example, persistent popliteal obstruction after DVT predicts the severity of postthrombotic chronic venous manifestations.[35]

Valvular destruction after DVT does not always occur, with only about half of thrombosed

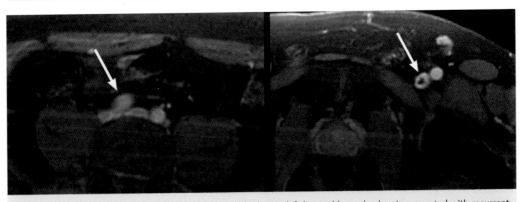

Fig. 2.7 May–Thurner anatomy. A 36-year-old man with chronic left leg and lower back pain presented with recurrent left lower extremity DVT. Left-hand panel: magnetic resonance angiogram (MRA) demonstrates severe compression of the left common iliac vein by the right common iliac artery (arrow). Right-hand panel: more inferior image demonstrates associated thrombus in the left external iliac vein (arrow).

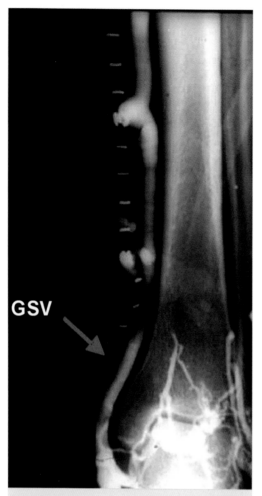

Fig. 2.8 Venogram of the distal right lower extremity demonstrating a dilated incompetent great saphenous vein (GSV).

segments demonstrating reflux 1 year after the DVT.[36] Interestingly, thrombus does not usually involve the valve cusps, and is separated from them possibly by valvular endothelial fibrinolytic mechanisms.[10] It is possible that thrombus initially adheres to the valves during the acute DVT episode, accounting for the later histologic features of postthrombotic syndrome, though more work is needed to elucidate the pathogenesis of valvular dysfunction after DVT.

2.4.4 Special Conditions

It is accepted that pregnancy significantly increases risk of CVI. Both overall increased blood volume and upstream obstruction by the gravid uterus impeding blood return to the heart play important roles.[9] During pregnancy, lower extremity veins dilate and demonstrate increasing reflux over the course of gestation, with effects more pronounced in the superficial venous system.[37] Interestingly, the development of varicose veins precedes increasing blood volume and mass effect by the uterus.[9] Thus, hormonal influences may play an important role, as mentioned previously.

It is well documented that obesity is a significant risk factor for CVI, and as mentioned earlier, this may relate to elevated proximal/central venous pressures. Interestingly, while the severity of lower extremity symptoms classic for venous disease increases with increasing obesity, in the majority of these patients, there is no anatomic evidence of underlying venous disease.[38] These findings suggest that obesity independently causes symptoms and signs similar to those caused by CVI. Also, ulcers in obese patients take longer to heal than other CVI patients and tend to recur more frequently.[38] More work is needed to elucidate how obesity and CVI interact.

A number of hereditary factors also play a role in the pathogenesis of CVI. Epidemiologic studies indicate a strong genetic component, with 70 to 80% of patients with CVI reporting an associated family history,[39] with some studies suggesting a multifactorial inheritance.[40] While further work is needed to elucidate which genes are involved in predisposing to CVI, likely targets include pathways involved in collagen and ECM modulation.[41]

In summary, symptomatic lower extremity varicose veins may develop as a result of alterations in the superficial or deep venous systems. Lower extremity venous pressure is determined by the balance of arterial inflow and venous outflow, which is in turn determined by the pump function of the lower extremity muscles and the structural integrity of the vein wall and ECM. Furthermore, more central obstructive lesions may cause venous hypertension and consequently venous insufficiency. Understanding anatomic patterns of venous disease is critical in localizing which vessels are involved, which will appropriately guide therapy.

References

[1] Khilnani NM, Grassi CJ, Kundu S, et al. Cardiovascular Interventional Radiological Society of Europe, American College of Phlebology, and Society of Interventional Radiology Standards of Practice Committees. Multi-society consensus quality

improvement guidelines for the treatment of lower-extremity superficial venous insufficiency with endovenous thermal ablation from the Society of Interventional Radiology, Cardiovascular Interventional Radiological Society of Europe, American College of Phlebology and Canadian Interventional Radiology Association. J Vasc Interv Radiol. 2010; 21(1):14–31

[2] Meissner MH, Gloviczki P, Bergan J, et al. Primary chronic venous disorders. J Vasc Surg. 2007; 46 Suppl S:54S–67S

[3] Alexander CJ. The epidemiology of varicose veins. Med J Aust. 1972; 1(5):215–218

[4] Beebe-Dimmer JL, Pfeifer JR, Engle JS, Schottenfeld D. The epidemiology of chronic venous insufficiency and varicose veins. Ann Epidemiol. 2005; 15(3):175–184

[5] Callam MJ. Epidemiology of varicose veins. Br J Surg. 1994; 81(2):167–173

[6] Nicholls SC. Sequelae of untreated venous insufficiency. Semin Intervent Radiol. 2005; 22(3):162–168

[7] Quinlan DJ, Alikhan R, Gishen P, Sidhu PS. Variations in lower limb venous anatomy: implications for US diagnosis of deep vein thrombosis. Radiology. 2003; 228(2):443–448

[8] Lim CS, Davies AH. Pathogenesis of primary varicose veins. Br J Surg. 2009; 96(11):1231–1242

[9] Goldman MP, Weiss RA, Bergan JJ. Diagnosis and treatment of varicose veins: a review. J Am Acad Dermatol. 1994; 31(3, Pt 1):393–413, quiz 414–416

[10] Meissner MH. Lower extremity venous anatomy. Semin Intervent Radiol. 2005; 22(3):147–156

[11] Meissner MH, Moneta G, Burnand K, et al. The hemodynamics and diagnosis of venous disease. J Vasc Surg. 2007; 46 Suppl S:4S–24S

[12] Araki CT, Back TL, Padberg FT, et al. The significance of calf muscle pump function in venous ulceration. J Vasc Surg. 1994; 20(6):872–877, discussion 878–879

[13] Labropoulos N, Giannoukas AD, Nicolaides AN, Veller M, Leon M, Volteas N. The role of venous reflux and calf muscle pump function in nonthrombotic chronic venous insufficiency. Correlation with severity of signs and symptoms. Arch Surg. 1996; 131(4):403–406

[14] Moneta GL, Nehler MR. The lower extremity venous system: anatomy and physiology of normal venous function and chronic venous insufficiency. In: Gloviczki P, Tao JST, eds. Handbook of Venous Disorders. Guidelines of the American Venous Forum. London: Chapman & Hall Medical; 1996:3–26

[15] Delis KT. Leg perforator vein incompetence: functional anatomy. Radiology. 2005; 235(1):327–334

[16] Somjen GM. Anatomy of the superficial venous system. Dermatol Surg. 1995; 21(1):35–45

[17] Gloviczki P, Mozes G. Development and anatomy of the venous system. In: Gloviczki P, ed. Handbook of Venous Disorders: Guidelines of the American Venous Forum. 3rd ed. Boca Raton, FL: CRC Press; 2008:12–36

[18] Thomson H. The surgical anatomy of the superficial and perforating veins of the lower limb. Ann R Coll Surg Engl. 1979; 61(3):198–205

[19] Mozes G, Gloviczki P, Menawat SS, Fisher DR, Carmichael SW, Kadar A. Surgical anatomy for endoscopic subfascial division of perforating veins. J Vasc Surg. 1996; 24(5):800–808

[20] Caggiati A, Bergan JJ, Gloviczki P, Jantet G, Wendell-Smith CP, Partsch H, International Interdisciplinary Consensus Committee on Venous Anatomical Terminology. Nomenclature of the veins of the lower limbs: an international interdisciplinary consensus statement. J Vasc Surg. 2002; 36(2):416–422

[21] Browse NL, Burnand KG, Thomas ML. Diseases of the Veins: Pathology, Diagnosis, and Treatment. London: Edward Arnold; 1988

[22] Smith RK, Golledge J. A systematic review of circulating markers in primary chronic venous insufficiency. Phlebology. 2014; 29(9):570–579

[23] Goodrich SM, Wood JE. The effect of estradiol-17-beta on peripheral venous distensibility and velocity of venous blood flow. Am J Obstet Gynecol. 1966; 96(3):407–412

[24] Meendering JR, Torgrimson BN, Houghton BL, Halliwill JR, Minson CT. Effects of menstrual cycle and oral contraceptive use on calf venous compliance. Am J Physiol Heart Circ Physiol. 2005; 288(1):H103–H110

[25] Kelechi TJ, Haight BK, Herman J, Michel Y, Brothers T, Edlund B. Skin temperature and chronic venous insufficiency. J Wound Ostomy Continence Nurs. 2003; 30(1):17–24

[26] Vanhoutte PM, Corcaud S, de Montrion C. Venous disease: from pathophysiology to quality of life. Angiology. 1997; 48 (7):559–567

[27] Stücker M, Steinbrügge J, Memmel U, Avermaete A, Altmeyer P. Disturbed vasomotion in chronic venous insufficiency. J Vasc Surg. 2003; 38(3):522–527

[28] Meissner MH, Eklof B, Smith PC, et al. Secondary chronic venous disorders. J Vasc Surg. 2007; 46 Suppl S:68S–83S

[29] Raju S, Neglén P. Clinical practice. Chronic venous insufficiency and varicose veins. N Engl J Med. 2009; 360 (22):2319–2327

[30] Masuda EM, Kistner RL. Long-term results of venous valve reconstruction: a four- to twenty-one-year follow-up. J Vasc Surg. 1994; 19(3):391–403

[31] Bergan JJ, Schmid-Schönbein GW, Smith PD, Nicolaides AN, Boisseau MR, Eklof B. Chronic venous disease. N Engl J Med. 2006; 355(5):488–498

[32] Ono T, Bergan JJ, Schmid-Schönbein GW, Takase S. Monocyte infiltration into venous valves. J Vasc Surg. 1998; 27(1):158–166

[33] Oklu R, Habito R, Mayr M, et al. Pathogenesis of varicose veins. J Vasc Interv Radiol. 2012; 23(1):33–39, quiz 40

[34] Sansilvestri-Morel P, Rupin A, Badier-Commander C, et al. Imbalance in the synthesis of collagen type I and collagen type III in smooth muscle cells derived from human varicose veins. J Vasc Res. 2001; 38(6):560–568

[35] Meissner MH, Caps MT, Zierler BK, et al. Determinants of chronic venous disease after acute deep venous thrombosis. J Vasc Surg. 1998; 28(5):826–833

[36] Markel A, Manzo RA, Bergelin RO, Strandness DE, Jr. Valvular reflux after deep vein thrombosis: incidence and time of occurrence. J Vasc Surg. 1992; 15(2):377–382, discussion 383–384

[37] Sparey C, Haddad N, Sissons G, Rosser S, de Cossart L. The effect of pregnancy on the lower-limb venous system of women with varicose veins. Eur J Vasc Endovasc Surg. 1999; 18(4):294–299

[38] Padberg F, Jr, Cerveira JJ, Lal BK, Pappas PJ, Varma S, Hobson RW, II. Does severe venous insufficiency have a different etiology in the morbidly obese? Is it venous? J Vasc Surg. 2003; 37(1):79–85

[39] Merlen JF, Coget J, Larère J. Heredity of varices [in French]. Phlebologie. 1967; 20(3):213–216

[40] Hauge M, Gundersen J. Genetics of varicose veins of the lower extremities. Hum Hered. 1969; 19(5):573–580

[41] Serra R, Buffone G, de Franciscis A, et al. A genetic study of chronic venous insufficiency. Ann Vasc Surg. 2012; 26 (5):636–642

3 Clinical Exam

Michael G. Johnson, Jr., Igor Rafael Sincos, and Felipe B. Collares

3.1 Introduction

The Society for Interventional Radiology, Cardiovascular Interventional Radiological Society of Europe, American College of Phlebology, Canadian Interventional Radiology Association, the Society for Vascular Surgery, and the American Venous Forum have developed quality improvement and clinical practice guidelines which recommend a complete history and a detailed physical examination for patients with varicose veins or chronic venous disease (CVD).[1,2,3] The initial clinical evaluation is an essential assessment that helps guide the management of patients with venous insufficiency. As a health care practitioner, it is important to provide a thorough examination keeping in mind that some patients referred for venous insufficiency may also suffer from other medical conditions that share similar clinical manifestations. In these situations, proper recognition of other conditions is necessary to direct the patient toward appropriate medical care. For those with venous insufficiency, the clinical exam will help the practitioner select the type of treatment and manage patient expectations appropriately. The postoperative evaluation is equally as important and used to determine if there has been improvement in symptoms or appearance of the legs, gauge patient satisfaction, and look for procedure-related complications. Both the pre- and postoperative assessments require a methodical, organized examination.

The proper function of the venous system of the lower extremities relies on one-way valves located at intervals along the course of the vessels keeping the direction of blood flow toward the heart. When these valves fail, blood is allowed to flow in a retrograde direction, commonly described as venous reflux. As a consequence, venous hypertension develops in the territory drained by the vessel. CVD is the clinical entity that results from chronic venous hypertension.[4,5]

Chronic venous insufficiency is a heterogeneous medical condition associated with a wide clinical spectrum, ranging from simple cosmetic issues to severe and limiting symptoms including venous ulcerations. The incidence increases with age, is higher in women than men, and worsens with pregnancy.[1,2,3,4,5,6,7,8] The lower extremity venous system consists of a network of superficial and deep veins interconnected by perforator veins, and the severity of signs and symptoms correlates with the extension of venous insufficiency within the system.[7]

The majority of patients presenting with venous insufficiency have idiopathic disease of the vein wall, with subsequent valvular incompetence in the superficial veins leading to venous reflux (superficial venous insufficiency) and development of varicose veins.[1,2,3,4] Most cases of deep venous insufficiency have a nonthrombotic (primary) or postthrombotic (secondary) etiology.[7] It is estimated that 23% of adults have varicose veins in the United States, and 6% present with more advanced CVD with skin changes, edema, or ulcerations.[1] Varicosities can be considered a cosmetic problem with variable impact in the lifestyle of patients. However, varicose veins are a common cause of discomfort, pain, disability, and deterioration of quality of life.[1]

Symptoms related to varicose veins can be variable. Some patients may present with no symptoms, only concerned about the cosmetic appearance of the visible veins. Symptoms related to varicose veins include aching, pain, burning sensation, tingling, throbbing, heaviness, tiredness and fatigue, itching skin, muscle cramps, swelling, and restless legs. Although not specific, these symptoms suggest CVD, particularly if they are more significant by the end of the day and are relieved by resting, elevation of the legs, or use of compression stockings.[1]

The clinical exam is composed of a thorough medical history, physical examination, photographic documentation of visible findings, classification into the CEAP (clinical, etiology, anatomy, pathophysiology) system, assignment of a venous clinical severity score (VCSS), and determination of treatment options and clinical follow-up. Each part is described in detail in this chapter.

3.2 Medical History

The patient history is necessary to establish the etiology of venous insufficiency, as well as gauge the severity of the disease and the impact on the patient's quality of life. The latter two will help assess procedure outcomes. The patient history should be thorough and efficient. An efficient way to help obtain thorough histories is to have a

Initial Visit Questionnaire

Name:_____   Date:_____

Birthdate:_____   Age:_____

Primary Care Physician:_____
PCP Address:_____

    Were you referred here by your PCP? ☐ Yes   ☐ No

Insurance Plan and Number:_____

Current Problem

1. **Do you experience any of the following symptoms in your legs? (please check)**

    ☐ aching/pain
    Please rate this pain, 1 being painless, 10 being incredibly painful:____

    ☐ heaviness   ☐ numbness/tingling   ☐ tiredness/fatigue   ☐ itching/burning

    ☐ swollen ankles   ☐ leg cramps   ☐ restless legs ☐ throbbing   ☐ tenderness

    ☐ warm leg   ☐ red leg   ☐ abnormally large veins   ☐ other:_____

2. **Do you experience these symptoms in the right leg, left leg or both?**_____
    If on both sides, which leg is worse?_____

3. **How often do you have these symptoms?** ☐ Constantly   ☐ Most of the time
                                          ☐ Sometimes   ☐ Almost never/ Never

4. **Please mark the following areas with "x" on the drawings below:**

Symptomatic areas   Areas of Cosmetic Concern

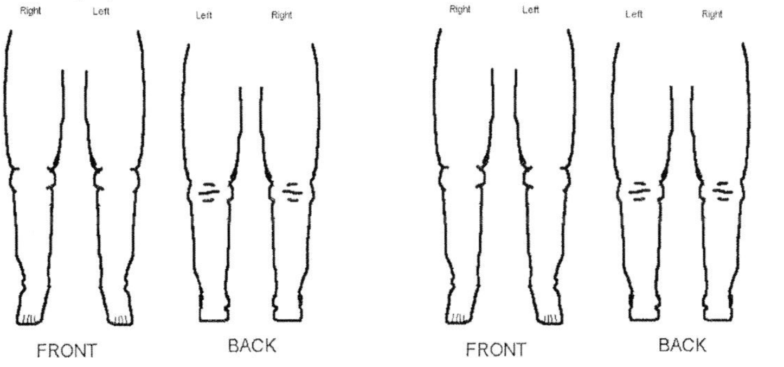

Right   Left   Left   Right   Right   Left   Left   Right

FRONT   BACK   FRONT   BACK

Fig. 3.1 Patient self-assessment questionnaire.

clinical questionnaire pertaining to venous insufficiency in the office (▶ Fig. 3.1) to be completed by the patient prior to the consult. Alternatively, the questionnaire can be mailed or e-mailed to the patient in advance. The following sections should be present on the questionnaire: chief complaint, history of present illness, past medical and surgical history, allergies, current medications, social

5. **How much do your symptoms restrict your activity?**
   ☐ I can do frequent vigorous exercise (running, heavy lifting, strenuous sports)
   ☐ I am limited to moderate activity (moving a table, vacuuming, bowling, golf)
   ☐ I can't do more than regular walking (short errands away from home) because of my vein symptoms
   ☐ I can only do occasional walking (room to room, going to mailbox) because of my vein symptoms
   ☐ I can hardly walk at all (mainly sit or lie down) because of my veins

6. **Have your veins gotten worse in recent months?** ☐ Yes   ☐ No
   IF YES, how much has your activity been reduced <u>in the past 4 weeks</u>?
   ☐ I can do frequent vigorous exercise (running, heavy lifting, strenuous sports)
   ☐ I am limited to moderate activity (moving a table, vacuuming, bowling, golf)
   ☐ I can't do more than regular walking (short errands away from home) because of my vein symptoms
   ☐ I can only do occasional walking (room to room, going to mailbox) because of my vein symptoms
   ☐ I can hardly walk at all (mainly sit or lie down) because of my veins

7. **Do you elevate your legs to relieve discomfort?**   ☐ Yes   ☐ No

8. **Do you wear compression stockings prescribed by your doctor?**   ☐ Yes   ☐ No

9. **Do you wear light support stockings (e.g. Sheer Energy)?**   ☐ Yes   ☐ No

10. **Do support or compression stockings provide relief?**   ☐ Yes   ☐ No   ☐ N/A

11. **Do you have any problem walking?**   ☐ Yes   ☐ No
    If so, how far can you walk? ☐ Not limited ☐ Greater than 5 blocks
    ☐ Less than 5 blocks ☐ Less than 1 block

12. **Do you stand much at home?** ☐ Yes   ☐ No   **at work?** ☐ Yes   ☐ No
    If so, how does standing affect your legs? _____

Past Medical History

13. **Venous History**
    Have you ever had your veins evaluated before? ☐ Yes   ☐ No
    If yes, when and where? _____

    Have you ever had any tests done on your veins? ☐ Yes   ☐ No
    If yes, please describe: _____

    Have you ever had vein stripping surgery? ☐ Yes   ☐ No
    If yes, when and which leg? _____

    Have you ever had vein injections? ☐ Yes   ☐ No
    If yes, when, where and which leg? _____

Fig. 3.1 (*continued*)

history, and family history. Pay particular attention to the risk factors in the history that will make venous disease more likely: older age, female gender, family history of venous insufficiency, obesity, occupation requiring prolonged standing or sitting, pregnancy, and previous deep venous thrombosis (DVT). Also pay attention to risk factors that would make another diagnosis more likely, such as

Have you ever had a blood clot? ☐ Yes   ☐ No
    If yes, which leg and when? _____

Have you ever had phlebitis? ☐ Yes   ☐ No
    If yes, which leg and when? _____

14. General Medical History
    Please list any hospitalizations you have had: _____
    _____

    Please list any surgeries you have had: _____
    _____

    Are you currently under the care of a physician? ☐ Yes   ☐ No
       If yes, for what illness or purpose? _____

    Do you have…
    ☐ heart disease   ☐ lung disease   ☐ high blood pressure   ☐ hepatitis
    ☐ arthritis   ☐ leg ulcer

15. Do you smoke? ☐ Yes   ☐ No
    If yes, how many packs per day? _____

16. Medications
    Do you take any blood-thinning medications? ☐ Yes   ☐ No   ☐ Not sure
    Do you take any hormones or birth control pills? ☐ Yes   ☐ No   ☐ Not sure

    Please list all the medications that you take:_____
    _____
    _____
    _____

17. Allergies
    Please list any allergies you have and describe the reaction: _____
    _____
    _____
    _____

18. Child-Rearing History
    Do you think you are currently pregnant? ☐ Yes   ☐ No
    Do you intend to have any more children? ☐ Yes   ☐ No
    How many times have you been pregnant? _____
    When was the last time you were pregnant? _____

19. Family History
    Has anyone in your family had varicose veins or spider veins?
    Father ☐ Yes   ☐ No   Mother ☐ Yes   ☐ No
    Brother(s) ☐ Yes   ☐ No   Sister(s) ☐ Yes   ☐ No
    Other(s):_____

Fig. 3.1 (*continued*)

peripheral arterial disease, lymphatic or deep venous obstruction, pelvic congestion syndrome, trauma, vasculitis, or infection.

3.2.1 History of Present Illness

Using the diagram of the legs in the questionnaire (► Fig. 3.1), have the patient mark the area(s) of concern on the front and back of the legs. The patient should specify the type of discomfort (heaviness, numbness/tingling, itching, burning, cramps, throbbing, tenderness, warmth, restlessness, etc.) and indicate the presence of visible findings such as redness, rash, skin discoloration, bulging veins, spider veins, swelling, or ulceration. The severity of each concern can be provided on a scale of 1 to 10. If it is a cosmetic concern, they should state what type and the location in the lower extremities.

These specific questions regarding the patient's symptoms are particularly useful:

- When does the pain occur? It is expected that pain related to venous insufficiency will occur after standing or sitting for long periods of time, and get worse throughout the day. If the pain is worse in the morning or when lying down, this should draw attention toward other etiologies. For example, rheumatoid arthritis affecting joints in the lower extremity may be painful in the morning, but improve throughout the day.[1] If there is pain or discomfort when lying down or at night, then consider restless leg syndrome, but be aware that there is an association between venous insufficiency and restless leg syndrome. Improvement of symptoms in these patients has been reported after the venous insufficiency has been successfully treated.[9] Whether the symptoms are constant or intermittent may depend on the intensity of physical activity during the day. The pain associated with venous insufficiency is expected to improve when the patient's legs are elevated and worsen with prolonged standing.[7,8]
- Do the patient's symptoms restrict his or her daily activities? If yes, and to a great extent, then consider that the patient may be experiencing claudication related to arterial insufficiency and peripheral vascular disease. Venous claudication (pain during and after exercise that is relieved with rest and leg elevation) can also be caused by venous outflow obstruction related to DVT or iliac vein stenosis (May–Thurner syndrome).[1]
- Have the symptoms been getting worse? Venous disease is expected to get worse over a period of months to years. If the symptoms started suddenly or are progressing rapidly, then other etiologies must also be considered.
- Has anything been done to improve the pain? Usually, the patient has tried leg elevation and maybe even compression stockings. If the patient has used compression stockings, then identify how often they have been worn and which type (over-the-counter vs. prescription). If prescription, check to see whether the graded compression of the stocking was appropriate for the patient's symptoms.

3.2.2 Past Medical and Surgical History

A thorough medical history should include past medical problems as well as previous surgical procedures. As part of the clinical assessment, it is particularly important to search for comorbidities that may preclude or increase the risk of venous interventions. Questions should address previous DVT or thrombophlebitis, history of thrombophilia, thrombotic disorders, vascular anomalies, peripheral vascular disease, and diabetes as well as previous surgical operations and procedures. Ask about known medical issues such as malignancy or recent operations or hospitalizations, which can increase the risk of DVT:

- Has this patient ever had his/her veins evaluated before and, if so, how long ago?
- Did the evaluation include an ultrasound assessment?
- Did the patient ever have treatment such as vein stripping, ablation, or sclerotherapy?
- Has the patient ever had phlebitis?
- If the patient is a female, ask if currently pregnant, if planning on future pregnancies, the number of previous pregnancies, and date of the last pregnancy. Conservative management with compression stockings and leg elevation is traditionally indicated if the patient is currently pregnant or considering pregnancy in the near future. Severe cases should be evaluated individually taking into consideration all risks and benefits of invasive treatment options.[8]

3.2.3 Family History

Ask the patient if family members have venous disease given that genetics have strongly been implicated in the development of venous insufficiency.[10] Varicose veins are thought to be autosomal dominant with incomplete penetrance, and when both parents have varicose veins, the offspring have a 90% chance of having them.[8,10,11]

3.2.4 Social History

Occupations that involve standing or sitting for prolonged periods of time can exacerbate venous disease.[7,8] Obesity and sedentariness are also risk factors for venous insufficiency.[1] It is reasonable to ask if the patient had any recent travel or has plans to travel, which has implications for when to treat. It is advisable to avoid elective invasive treatments prior to a long flight due to increased risk for DVT. Explain to the patient that physical activity (ambulation) should be encouraged following invasive treatments to reduce chances of DVT.[12] Furthermore, a positive history of tobacco, alcohol, or recreational drug use can suggest the presence of important comorbidities.

3.2.5 Allergies

All known allergies should be revealed. Ask if the patient is allergic to lidocaine, latex, or chemical sclerosants such as Sotradecol or polidocanol given that these may be used during venous interventions. Although rare, allergic reactions and anaphylaxis after injection of sclerosing agents can occur.[1]

3.2.6 Medications

- *Oral contraceptives*: They are known risk factors for DVT.[13]
- *Anticoagulation*: There is no evidence to support the routine use of anticoagulation for thrombosis prophylaxis prior to or after endovenous thermal ablation (EVTA) procedures.[3] On the other hand, EVTA can be safely performed in patients with chronic venous insufficiency requiring long-term warfarin therapy without discontinuation of anticoagulation.[14]

3.3 Physical Examination

The physical examination should start with the patient standing in a warm room with good illumination. The clinical evaluation should focus on visible signs of venous disease, which can be helpful in determining the anatomic pattern of venous insufficiency. Physical examination findings such as size, location, and distribution of enlarged veins should be documented, and may include photographs. The physician should pay particular attention to the patient's ankle because this is probably the most vulnerable region for skin changes and ulcers. Inspection and palpation are essential parts of the physical examination, and auscultation may be helpful in cases of vascular malformations of arteriovenous fistulae, on which a bruit can be noticed.

There are several findings on physical exam unrelated to venous insufficiency that can mimic venous disease. These findings range from relatively benign such as lipomas and bruising to more concerning findings such as infections, lymphadenopathy, melanoma, or other skin cancers. These should be taken into consideration to promote appropriate medical care.

3.3.1 Physical Manifestations of Venous Disease[1,7,15]

Inspection

- *Telangiectasias*: a confluence of small dilated intradermal blood vessels of less than 1 mm in caliber. Synonyms include spider veins, hyphen webs, and thread veins.
- *Corona phlebectatica*: fan-shaped pattern of numerous small intradermal veins commonly seen around the medial or lateral aspects of the ankle and foot.
- *Reticular veins*: dilated intradermal veins, usually of blue color, measuring from 1 mm to less than 3 mm in diameter.
- *Varicose veins*: subcutaneous dilated and tortuous veins measuring more than 3 mm in diameter with the patient in standing position. Varicose veins develop as a result of valvular incompetence and may involve saphenous veins, saphenous tributaries, or nonsaphenous veins.
  - When evaluating varicosities, look for patterns of disease:
    - a) *Medial thigh and/or calf*: great saphenous vein reflux.
    - b) *Anterior thigh*: anterior accessory saphenous vein.
    - c) *Groin or vulvar varicosities*: pelvic congestion syndrome (ovarian vein reflux).
    - d) *Posterior upper thigh*: inferior gluteal vein reflux.[16]
- *Edema*: increase in volume of extravascular fluid in the subcutaneous tissue and skin, usually more evident in the ankle region, but may extend to the leg and foot.
- *Venous stasis dermatitis/venous eczema*: erythematous dermatitis (red rash or brown

discoloration) that develops as a result of increased pressure in the capillary bed, which the patient may describe as itchy. It can be present anywhere in the lower extremity but is often located in the lower leg, around the ankle, or near varicose veins.[1,17]

- *Hyperpigmentation*: dark brownish discoloration of the skin, which usually occurs in the lower leg and ankle regions.
- *Lipodermatosclerosis*: discolored scarred skin associated with severe CVD. In addition to hyperpigmentation, cutaneous sclerosis or scarring has occurred.
- *Ulceration*: skin defect that usually occurs over the medial malleolus and can be seen in healing or active phases.

Palpation

Palpate for cords, varicosities, pitting edema, tenderness, induration, reflux, thrill, groin, or abdominal masses. Also, examine the arterial pulses in the leg, knee, and foot to evaluate for possible arterial insufficiency.

3.4 Imaging

For a complete assessment, the medical history and physical exam should always be supplemented by ultrasound evaluation of the lower extremities (Chapter 4). For patients with varicose veins and more advanced CVD, computed tomography venography, magnetic resonance venography, ascending and descending contrast venography, and intravascular ultrasonography should be used selectively for conditions such as postthrombotic syndrome, thrombotic or nonthrombotic iliac vein obstruction (May–Thurner syndrome), pelvic congestion syndrome, nutcracker syndrome, vascular malformations, venous trauma, and tumors, and to plan complex open or endovascular venous interventions.[1]

3.5 Classification and Quality-of-Life Assessment

CVD has been classified by various systems, which allow researchers to communicate their diagnosis and assess treatment outcomes.[15,18,19,20,21,22,23,24,25] The subjective and objective findings gathered from the history and physical exam can be organized using disease-specific severity scoring models such as the CEAP classification[15] and the VCSS[18,19,20] (▶ Fig. 3.2). It has also been suggested that a

disease-specific quality-of-life questionnaire be used.[1] In this section, we briefly describe the 20-item chronic venous insufficiency quality-of-life questionnaire (CIVIQ-20),[23] a quality-of-life questionnaire that has been validated for use in the United States and in other countries.[24,25]

3.5.1 CEAP

The Society for Vascular Surgery and the American Venous Forum recommend that the CEAP classification be used for all patients with CVD.[1] The CEAP system was created to classify CVD by its clinical characteristics, etiologic factors, anatomic distributions, and underlying pathophysiologic factors in a way that standardizes physician observations for treatment and outcome comparison.[15]

Clinical Classification

- C0: no evidence of venous disease.
- C1: presence of telangiectasias or reticular veins only.
- C2: presence of varicose veins.
- C3: presence of edema.
- C4: Presence of skin changes:
  - C4a: presence of pigmentation or eczema.
  - C4b: presence of lipodermatosclerosis.
- C5: presence of healed venous ulcer.
- C6: presence of active venous ulcer.

Etiologic Classification

- Ec: congenital etiology.
- Ep: primary etiology.
- Es: secondary (postthrombotic) etiology.
- En: no venous etiology identified.

Anatomic Classification

- As: superficial venous system.
- Ap: perforator veins.
- Ad: deep venous system.
- An: no venous location identified.

Pathophysiologic Classification

- Pr: reflux.
- Po: obstruction.
- Pro: reflux and obstruction.
- Pn: no venous pathophysiology identifiable.

As an example, the CEAP classification for the patient shown in ▶ Fig. 3.2a is C4a Ep As Pr. The

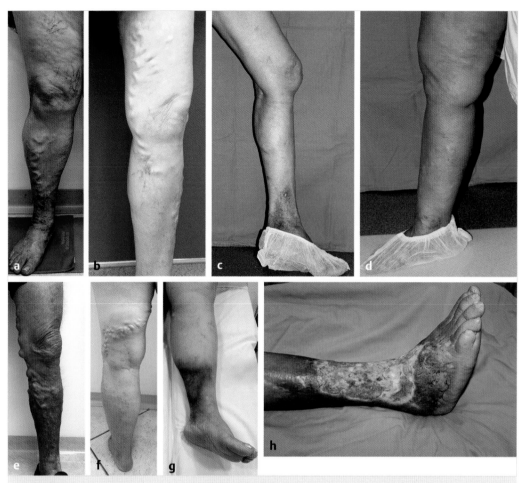

Fig. 3.2 Examples of patients with chronic venous insufficiency with respective CEAP classifications and venous clinical severity scores (VCSSs). The VCSSs include the following elements: pain or discomfort; varicose veins (VV); edema; skin pigmentation; inflammation; induration; number of active ulcers; active ulcer size; and use of compression therapy (Comp). **(a)** Pain = 2; VV = 2; edema = 1; pigmentation = 2; inflammation = 0; induration = 0; ulcer number = 0; ulcer size = 0; Comp = 2; CEAP = C4a; VCSS = 9. **(b)** Pain = 1; VV = 3; edema = 1; pigmentation = 0; inflammation = 0; induration = 0; ulcer number = 0; ulcer size = 0; Comp = 1; CEAP= C3; VCSS= 6. **(c)** Pain = 1; VV = 1; edema = 0; pigmentation = 1; inflammation = 0; induration = 0; ulcer number = 0; ulcer size = 0; Comp = 2; CEAP= C5; VCSS= 5. **(d)** Pain = 2; VV = 1; edema = 2; pigmentation = 0; inflammation = 0; induration = 0; ulcer number = 0; ulcer size = 0; Comp = 1; CEAP= C3; VCSS= 6. **(e)** Pain = 1; VV = 3; edema = 2; pigmentation = 3; inflammation = 2; induration = 1; ulcer number = 0; ulcer size = 0; Comp = 1; CEAP = C4b; VCSS = 13. **(f)** Pain = 1; VV = 2; edema = 1; pigmentation = 2; inflammation = 0; induration = 0; ulcer number = 0; ulcer size = 0; Comp = 1; CEAP= 3; VCSS= 7. **(g)** Pain = 3; VV = 2; edema = 2; pigmentation = 3; inflammation = 2; induration = 2; ulcer number = 0; ulcer size = 0; Comp = 2; CEAP= 5; VCSS= 16. **(h)** Pain = 3; VV = 2; edema = 2; pigmentation = 3; inflammation = 3; induration = 3; ulcer number = 2; ulcer size = 3; Comp = 1; CEAP= 6; VCSS= 22.

advanced CEAP is the same basic classification with the inclusion of 18 named venous segments that can be used as locators for venous pathology:

- Superficial veins:
  1. Telangiectasias/reticular veins.
  2. Great saphenous vein above knee.
  3. Great saphenous vein below knee.
  4. Small saphenous vein.
  5. Nonsaphenous veins.
- Deep veins:
  1. Inferior vena cava.
  2. Common iliac vein.
  3. Internal iliac vein.
  4. External iliac vein.

5. Pelvic: gonadal, broad ligament veins, other.
6. Common femoral vein.
7. Deep femoral vein.
8. Femoral vein.
9. Popliteal vein.
10. Crural: anterior tibial, posterior tibial, fibular veins.
11. Muscular: gastrocnemial, soleal veins, other.

- Perforating veins:
  1. Thigh.
  2. Calf.

3.5.2 The Venous Clinical Severity Score

The VCSS is a quality-of-life tool that supplements the CEAP classification.[18,19,20,21,22] The Society for Vascular Surgery and the American Venous Forum recommend that the VCSS be used to assess outcomes for patients with CVD.[1,20] It is particularly useful for grading severe manifestations of chronic venous insufficiency in patients described as CEAP clinical C2 or higher, even more so for severe cases, such as CEAP classification C4 to C6. The use of this scoring system reduces intraobserver and interobserver variability, allowing for better outcomes assessment with more accurate comparison of patients signs and symptoms before and after treatment.[18,19,20,21,22]

The VCSS includes nine important elements (signs and symptoms) of venous disease, each scored on a severity scale from 0 to 3 (0 = absence of sign or symptom; 1 = mild; 2 = moderate; and 3 = severe). The revised version also includes the use of compression therapy[20]:

- *Pain or discomfort*: 0 = none; 1 = mild discomfort or occasional pain; 2 = daily pain interfering but not limiting daily activities; 3 = severe, limiting pain.
- *Varicose veins*: 0 = none; 1 = few, scattered; 2 = confined to calf or thigh; 3 = involves both calf and thigh.
- *Edema*: 0 = none; 1 = limited to foot and ankle; 2 = below the knee; 3 = extension above the knee.
- *Skin pigmentation*: 0 = none; 1 = limited to perimalleolar area; 2 = diffuse on the lower third of the calf; 3 = extension above the lower third of the calf.
- *Inflammation* (dermatitis, eczema): 0 = none; 1 = limited to perimalleolar area; 2 = diffuse on the lower third of the calf; 3 = extension above the lower third of the calf.
- *Induration* (lipodermatosclerosis): 0 = none; 1 = limited to perimalleolar area; 2 = diffuse on the lower third of the calf; 3 = extension above the lower third of the calf
- *Number of active ulcers*: 0; 1; 2; 3 (for three or more ulcers).
- *Active ulcer duration*: 0 = no ulcer; 1 = less than 3 months; 2 = more than 3 months but less than 1 year; 3 = more than 1 year without healing.
- *Active ulcer size*: 0 = no ulcer; 1 = diameter less than 2 cm; 2 = diameter between 2 and 6 cm; 3 = diameter of more than 6 cm.
- *Use of compression therapy*: 0 = no use; 1 = occasional use; 2 = frequent use; 3 = daily use or full compliance.

3.5.3 The CIVIQ-20

The CIVIQ-20 is a 20-item self-reported quality-of-life questionnaire that was created and validated in France in 1996.[23] It has been translated into 13 languages and validated for use in 18 countries, including the United States.[24,25,26] The questionnaire includes four dimensions: physical (four items), psychologic (nine items), social (three items), and pain (four items). An electronic copy of the CIVIQ-20 can be obtained on the CIVIQ-20 website (www.civiq-20.com). This questionnaire is a disease-specific instrument with good consistency and reliability and high sensitivity to changes in the quality of life in patients that improved clinically after treatment.[27]

3.6 Photographic Documentation

With the patient's permission, perform photographic documentation to monitor the progress of treatment and final outcome. Photos should be taken at the first consult or before the first venous intervention. Ideally, before and after comparisons should be obtained with the same camera, position, angle, and lighting. Most of the digital cameras on the market today provide sufficient resolution for the necessary imaging; however, since photo quality, printers, and displays vary, always make comparisons between photos, rather than between the patient and a photo. Taking pictures and comparing before and after photos requires some equipment and training. It is a task that does not need to be done by the physician, but should be done each time with a similar protocol and equipment.

Suggested photo-documentation protocol:
- Digital single-lens reflex (DSLR) camera.
- Standardized room and camera light sources.
- Standardized camera settings according to equipment and room.
- Standardized camera and patient positioning with the camera perpendicular to the skin.
- Obtain panoramic pictures of the lower extremities.
- Obtain spot pictures of relevant findings.

Frequently transfer the photos to a secure patient file folder on your office computer for future reference. Thorough photographic documentation serves as an important quality assurance or quality improvement tool, as well as for medicolegal documentation.

3.7 Managing Patient Expectations

Patients with visible or enlarged veins in the lower extremities will often seek medical attention for two main reasons: symptom relief and cosmetic improvement. Symptoms related to venous insufficiency are variable and may not correlate with the visible findings or the degree and extent of disease. The cosmetic appearance of the visible veins can produce a significant psychologic impact on patients, affecting their lifestyle and overall quality of life.[1] Patients seeking cosmetic treatment may have a history of unsuccessful procedures or unsatisfactory results due to underlying venous reflux that has not been appropriately worked up and treated.

Good communication with the patient is paramount. It is important to explain the nature of venous reflux in lay terms. A useful analogy is the concept of a leaking pipe (incompetent saphenous vein) that causes a stain on the wall (varicosities and visible veins). Painting the wall will not prevent recurrence of the stain if the plumbing is not repaired—similarly, cosmetic and symptom improvements will be suboptimal if the underlying venous insufficiency is left untreated. Patients should be aware that most treatments, for medical or cosmetic reasons, may require multiple interventions or sessions for the desired outcome. The planned interventions should also be described in simple terms for full understanding. All risks and benefits of procedures should be addressed and documented on a written informed consent form.

Patients should know what to expect on the immediate postprocedure period, to decrease anxiety and avoid unnecessary stress. They must also be aware that compliance with postprocedure care, such as the use of compression stockings, can have a direct impact on results. When comparing before and after images, do everything possible to control variables between photos. As mentioned in the photographic documentation section, compare photos taken using the same camera, position, and lighting on similar displays, if possible. Measurement and comparisons of clinical outcomes can be performed with the use of the VCSS and disease-specific quality-of-life questionnaires.

In conclusion, the discussion regarding the patient's clinical condition, treatment options, and possible outcomes should be open and honest, in order to create realistic expectations for symptom relief and cosmetic improvement.

References

[1] Gloviczki P, Comerota AJ, Dalsing MC, et al. Society for Vascular Surgery, American Venous Forum. The care of patients with varicose veins and associated chronic venous diseases: clinical practice guidelines of the Society for Vascular Surgery and the American Venous Forum. J Vasc Surg. 2011; 53(5) Suppl:2S–48S

[2] Kundu S, Grassi CJ, Khilnani NM, et al. Cardiovascular Interventional Radiological Society of Europe, American College of Phlebology, and Society of Interventional Radiology Standards of Practice Committees. Multi-disciplinary quality improvement guidelines for the treatment of lower extremity superficial venous insufficiency with ambulatory phlebectomy from the Society of Interventional Radiology, Cardiovascular Interventional Radiological Society of Europe, American College of Phlebology and Canadian Interventional Radiology Association. J Vasc Interv Radiol. 2010; 21(1):1–13

[3] Khilnani NM, Grassi CJ, Kundu S, et al. Cardiovascular Interventional Radiological Society of Europe, American College of Phlebology, and Society of Interventional Radiology Standards of Practice Committees. Multi-society consensus quality improvement guidelines for the treatment of lower-extremity superficial venous insufficiency with endovenous thermal ablation from the Society of Interventional Radiology, Cardiovascular Interventional Radiological Society of Europe, American College of Phlebology and Canadian Interventional Radiology Association. J Vasc Interv Radiol. 2010; 21(1):14–31

[4] Kouri B. Current evaluation and treatment of lower extremity varicose veins. Am J Med. 2009; 122(6):513–515

[5] Nicolaides AN, Hussein MK, Szendro G, Christopoulos D, Vasdekis S, Clarke H. The relation of venous ulceration with ambulatory venous pressure measurements. J Vasc Surg. 1993; 17(2):414–419

[6] Meissner MH, Gloviczki P, Bergan J, et al. Primary chronic venous disorders. J Vasc Surg. 2007; 46 Suppl S:54S–67S

[7] Raju S, Neglén P. Clinical practice. Chronic venous insufficiency and varicose veins. N Engl J Med. 2009; 360 (22):2319–2327

[8] Hamdan A. Management of varicose veins and venous insufficiency. JAMA. 2012; 308(24):2612–2621

[9] Langer RD, Ho E, Denenberg JO, Fronek A, Allison M, Criqui MH. Relationships between symptoms and venous disease: the San Diego population study. Arch Intern Med. 2005; 165 (12):1420–1424

[10] Pistorius MA. Chronic venous insufficiency: the genetic influence. Angiology. 2003; 54 Suppl 1:S5–S12

[11] Cornu-Thenard A, Boivin P, Baud JM, De Vincenzi I, Carpentier PH. Importance of the familial factor in varicose disease. Clinical study of 134 families. J Dermatol Surg Oncol. 1994; 20 (5):318–326

[12] Vedantham S. Superficial venous interventions: assessing the risk of DVT. Phlebology. 2008; 23(2):53–57

[13] Vandenbroucke JP, Rosing J, Bloemenkamp KW, et al. Oral contraceptives and the risk of venous thrombosis. N Engl J Med. 2001; 344(20):1527–1535

[14] Delaney CL, Russell DA, Iannos J, Spark JI. Is endovenous laser ablation possible while taking warfarin? Phlebology. 2012; 27(5):231–234

[15] Eklöf B, Rutherford RB, Bergan JJ, et al. American Venous Forum International Ad Hoc Committee for Revision of the CEAP Classification. Revision of the CEAP classification for chronic venous disorders: consensus statement. J Vasc Surg. 2004; 40(6):1248–1252

[16] Jiang P, van Rij AM, Christie RA, Hill GB, Thomson IA. Non-saphenofemoral venous reflux in the groin in patients with varicose veins. Eur J Vasc Endovasc Surg. 2001; 21(6):550–557

[17] Sippel K, Mayer D, Ballmer B, et al. Evidence that venous hypertension causes stasis dermatitis. Phlebology. 2011; 26 (8):361–365

[18] Rutherford RB, Padberg FT, Jr, Comerota AJ, Kistner RL, Meissner MH, Moneta GL. Venous severity scoring: an adjunct to venous outcome assessment. J Vasc Surg. 2000; 31(6):1307–1312

[19] Ricci MA, Emmerich J, Callas PW, et al. Evaluating chronic venous disease with a new venous severity scoring system. J Vasc Surg. 2003; 38(5):909–915

[20] Vasquez MA, Rabe E, McLafferty RB, et al. American Venous Forum Ad Hoc Outcomes Working Group. Revision of the venous clinical severity score: venous outcomes consensus statement: special communication of the American Venous Forum Ad Hoc Outcomes Working Group. J Vasc Surg. 2010; 52(5):1387–1396

[21] Kakkos SK, Rivera MA, Matsagas MI, et al. Validation of the new venous severity scoring system in varicose vein surgery. J Vasc Surg. 2003; 38(2):224–228

[22] Meissner MH, Natiello C, Nicholls SC. Performance characteristics of the venous clinical severity score. J Vasc Surg. 2002; 36(5):889–895

[23] Launois R, Reboul-Marty J, Henry B. Construction and validation of a quality of life questionnaire in chronic lower limb venous insufficiency (CIVIQ). Qual Life Res. 1996; 5(6):539–554

[24] Launois R, Mansilha A, Jantet G. International psychometric validation of the Chronic Venous Disease quality of life Questionnaire (CIVIQ-20). Eur J Vasc Endovasc Surg. 2010; 40 (6):783–789

[25] Radak DJ, Vlajinac HD, Marinković JM, Maksimović MŽ, Maksimović ZV. Quality of life in chronic venous disease patients measured by short Chronic Venous Disease Quality of Life Questionnaire (CIVIQ-14) in Serbia. J Vasc Surg. 2013; 58 (4):1006–1013

[26] Launois R, Mansilha A, Lozano F. Linguistic validation of the 20 item-chronic venous disease quality-of-life questionnaire (CIVIQ-20). Phlebology. 2014; 29(7):484–487

[27] Vasquez MA, Munschauer CE. Venous Clinical Severity Score and quality-of-life assessment tools: application to vein practice. Phlebology. 2008; 23(6):259–275

4 Imaging

Cyrillo R. Araujo, Jr. and Felipe B. Collares

4.1 Lower Extremity Vein Mapping with Duplex Ultrasound

Duplex ultrasonography (duplex US) is a widely accepted initial imaging modality for evaluation of varicose vein disease in the legs. It is also the imaging method of choice in the assessment of recurrent varicose veins and chronic venous insufficiency.[1] The risk of recurrence of varicose vein disease is directly related to the accuracy of preoperative diagnosis and effective image-guided therapies.[2]

The variability of venous anatomy is high, with significant variations occurring in almost 25% of patients with uncomplicated varicose veins and even more frequently in recurrent disease.[3] Duplex US can noninvasively and accurately evaluate leg veins and provide crucial information about location, degree, and patterns of venous reflux. A schematic diagram of the whole leg displaying the duplex US findings (duplex mapping) is essential for treatment planning in lower extremity venous disease. The example presented here is simple and offers a clear, comprehensible visual display of the venous anatomy and function in the leg, allowing the planning of appropriate therapy (▶ Fig. 4.1).

4.2 Basics of Venous Flow Dynamics

In normal circumstances, the superficial venous system drains the subcutaneous tissues and periodically empties into the deep system via perforating veins. Flow direction should always be cephalad and superficial to deep.

The veins contain a series of valves along their course, preventing retrograde flow back down the leg (▶ Fig. 4.2). If functioning properly, it is considered a competent valve. If blood is able to pass backward through the valve, it is deemed incompetent. Depending on the extent of incompetence, this backflow will fill the superficial veins, making them tortuous and dilated (varicose veins).

4.2.1 Duplex Ultrasound Examination for Venous Mapping

The duplex ultrasound examination for venous mapping should demonstrate both the anatomic

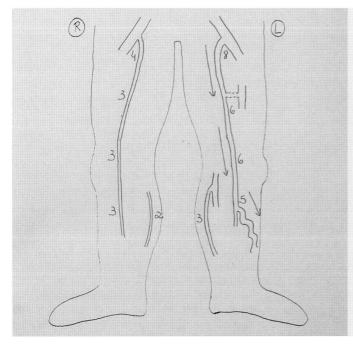

Fig. 4.1 Venous mapping worksheet. Example of a simple vein map of the lower extremities showing bilateral great and small saphenous veins. The numbers indicate the diameters of the veins at different levels in millimeters. Dotted lines represent a perforating vein in the left thigh, tortuous lines represent a varicose vein in the left calf, and arrows represent venous reflux in the left GSV.

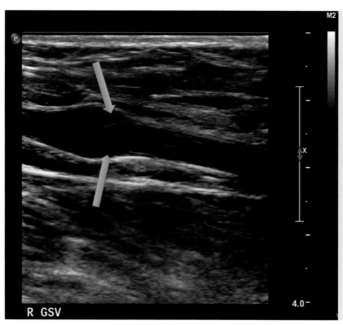

Fig. 4.2 Transverse ultrasound image of the great saphenous vein showing the venous valve (arrow).

R GSV

patterns of veins and abnormalities of venous blood flow in the lower extremities.[4] The following data should be recorded:

- Incompetent saphenous junctions, and their locations and diameters.
- The extent of reflux in the saphenous veins of the thighs and legs and their diameters.
- The number, location, diameter, and function of incompetent perforating veins.
- Other relevant veins that show reflux.
- The source of filling of all superficial varices if not from the veins already described.
- Veins that are hypoplastic, atretic, or absent, or that have been removed.
- The state of the deep venous system including competence of valves and evidence of previous venous thrombosis.

Most patients undergoing duplex ultrasound to investigate superficial, deep, and perforating veins are being considered for treatment of varicose veins. Information provided by the duplex mapping will usually have a significant impact on whether treatment will be offered and the type of treatment considered most appropriate.

Understanding the anatomy of the venous system is crucial to the correct evaluation and appropriate treatment of venous disorders. The veins of the lower extremities are divided into three systems: superficial, deep, and perforating venous systems. These are located in two main compartments: the superficial compartment and the deep compartment, which are, respectively, situated above and below the muscle fascia.

4.2.2 The Deep Veins

The deep veins are the primary route for returning blood to the heart. They collect the venous blood from all the draining muscular and superficial veins.

Ultrasound protocols usually include the following lower extremity deep veins[5]:

- Common femoral vein (CFV).
- Femoral vein (FV).
- Popliteal vein (POPV).
- Anterior tibial vein.
- Posterior tibial vein (PTV).
- Peroneal veins (PerVs).

4.2.3 The Superficial Veins

There are two main superficial veins draining the subcutaneous tissue of the lower extremity[6,7,8]:

- The great saphenous vein (GSV) runs from the medial malleolus, up the medial aspect of the leg and thigh, draining into the CFV at the groin through the saphenofemoral junction (SFJ).
- The small saphenous vein (SSV) runs up the posterior midline of the calf. It may drain into the proximal POPV above the knee crease as the saphenopopliteal junction (SPJ). Commonly, however, it may continue up the posterior thigh

as the Giacomini vein. This will terminate either into the mid/distal FV or ascend to drain into the proximal GSV.

- SFJ (▶ Fig. 4.3).
- The termination of the GSV into the CFV in the groin.

- It is the primary source of venous incompetence and varices of the lower extremity.
- SPJ (▶ Fig. 4.4).
- The termination of the SSV into the POPV in the popliteal fossa.

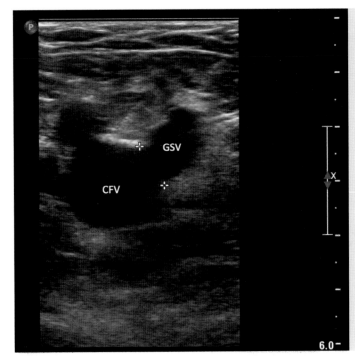

Fig. 4.3 Transverse ultrasound image at the level of the saphenofemoral (between " + " signs). It represents the confluence of the great saphenous vein (GSV) with the common femoral vein (CFV).

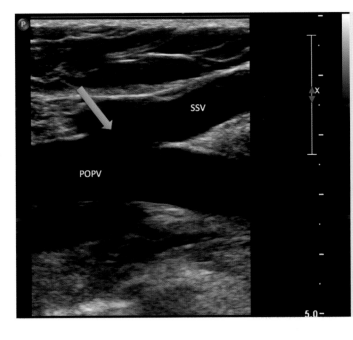

Fig. 4.4 Longitudinal ultrasound image at the level of the saphenopopliteal junction (arrow), representing the confluence of the small saphenous vein (SSV) with the popliteal vein (POPV).

- The SPJ is absent in 15 to 20% of the population, with the SSV continuing up posteriorly as the thigh extension of the SSV and Giacomini vein.[9]
- The SPJ is located in most cases (98%) in the upper lateral quadrant of the popliteal fossa. The remaining junctions are medial/lateral, often via a gastrocnemius vein.[10]

4.3 Doppler Ultrasound Exam

Duplex US is the primary diagnostic tool used to evaluate patients with superficial venous insufficiency. Duplex US is an inexpensive, portable, and reproducible means of simultaneously assessing both the venous anatomy and physiology.[11] As stated previously, duplex US can localize and specify the source of the venous problem to provide a map to help select the best treatment and evaluate outcome for the venous treatments (discussed later).

4.3.1 Indications for Duplex Scanning

As venous reflux commonly affects both lower extremities, it is advised that both extremities be scanned at the initial investigation, although this is dependent on the resources of the diagnostic service. The superficial and deep venous systems should be evaluated. The main indications are as follows[4,12,13,14,15,16]:

- Patients with uncomplicated great saphenous territory varicose veins.
- Patients with uncomplicated small saphenous territory varicose veins.
- Patients with nonsaphenous varicose veins (related to pelvic/perineal vein reflux or isolated lateral thigh varicose veins).
- Patients with recurrent varicose veins. Duplex scanning is considered to be essential to establish the complex anatomy and flow dynamics of recurrent varices to show whether surgery or endovenous treatment is appropriate.
- Patients with chronic venous disease with complications. Duplex scanning is considered to be essential to assess the involvement of the deep and superficial venous systems to predict the likely outcome after treating superficial disease alone and to select appropriate patients for deep venous reconstruction.
- Patients undergoing surveillance after treatment. This may be used to assess the outcome of therapy and for early detection of recurrence.

- Patients with venous malformations. Duplex US may be used initially to investigate and provide good management for vascular malformations. The investigation provides anatomic information about the extent of the malformation and its relationship to other vessels in the affected extremity. It may also be used to guide treatment of malformations by percutaneous therapy. It is frequently used before further investigation with magnetic resonance imaging and angiography.

4.3.2 Equipment Requirements and Settings

A color duplex ultrasound machine is required for this investigation.

A high-frequency linear array transducer of 7 to 12 MHz is appropriate for lower extremity investigation to obtain good quality images of the superficial veins. A curvilinear array transducer of 3.5 to 5 MHz can be useful for very large or edematous extremities.

B-mode Ultrasound Settings

Superficial veins normally lie 1 to 3 cm below the skin. They are usually imaged in the longitudinal view with the proximal end of the veins to the left of the screen, and in the transverse view with the lateral aspect of the right extremity and medial aspect of the left extremity shown to the left of the screen. The focal zone for the transducer should be set at an appropriate level to obtain the best B-mode image of the vein under investigation. Gain and dynamic gain control should be set to optimize the image so that the lumen of the vein should be dark (anechoic) in the absence of acute or chronic thrombosis and very slow flow, but to allow echoes from thrombus to be seen from within the lumen, when present.[4]

Pulsed-Wave Spectral or Color Doppler Settings

The use of slow flow settings is recommended to optimize the machine for slow velocities seen within veins. Set the Doppler range to 5 to 10 cm/s, with the wall filter at its lowest setting. It is best to increase the Doppler gain to show a small amount of "noise" in the color or pulsed Doppler signal to ensure maximum sensitivity of the system. It is advisable to increase the Doppler range and decrease the color gain in patients with high

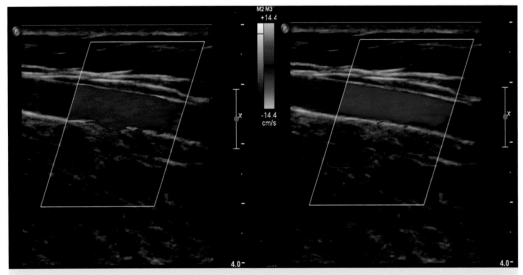

Fig. 4.5 Longitudinal ultrasound images of the great saphenous vein (GSV) at the level of the proximal thigh during (left image) and after augmentation (right image). Antegrade blood flow is represented in blue during augmentation followed by retrograde blood flow represented in red (venous reflux).

venous flow to avoid significant color artifact. It is conventional to use blue to represent antegrade venous flow toward the heart in the color mode and red for the reverse (venous reflux) direction (▶ Fig. 4.5).[4]

4.3.3 Patient Position and Ultrasound Probe

In general, it is recommended that examination of the superficial veins should be performed with the patient standing. The horizontal position is inappropriate for detection of reflux and measurement of vein diameters. However, both the lying and standing positions have been reported in the literature.[4]

Examination of calf veins can be performed with the patient in either the sitting or standing position (▶ Fig. 4.6). Transverse and longitudinal views of the veins should be employed in duplex ultrasound scanning of the lower extremities. The transverse view gives more precise general information regarding morphology and possible presence of endoluminal thrombus through the compression maneuver, while a longitudinal view helps to assess direction of flow and venous reflux more accurately. A Doppler angle of 45 to 60° between the transducer and vein should be used to achieve the optimum color or spectral Doppler signal (▶ Fig. 4.7).

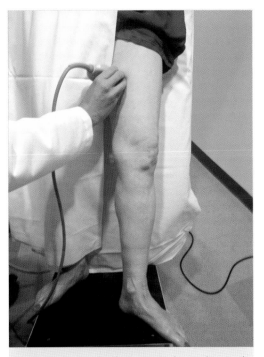

Fig. 4.6 Patient in standing position during ultrasound examination of the left lower extremity.

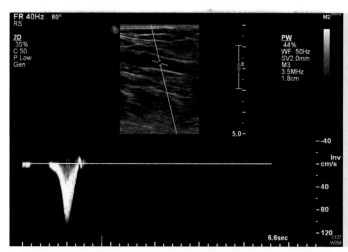

Fig. 4.7 Doppler ultrasound examination of a competent proximal great saphenous vein. Spectral waveform shows antegrade blood flow with no evidence of venous reflux.

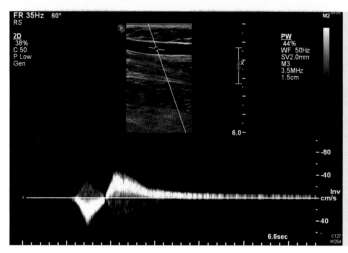

Fig. 4.8 Assessment of venous reflux with spectral Doppler ultrasound: antegrade flow in the proximal great saphenous vein is demonstrated during compression of the calf, followed by significant venous reflux.

4.4 Examination for Reflux: Based on the Venous Duplex Consensus[4,17,18]

4.4.1 Definition of Venous Reflux

Venous reflux is considered to be retrograde flow in the reverse direction to physiologic flow lasting for more than 0.5 s.[12] However, a definitive cutoff for all vein segments has not been agreed in the literature.

Different methods are used to elicit reflux:
- Release after a calf squeeze for proximal veins or foot squeeze for calf veins.
- Manual compression of vein clusters.
- Pneumatic calf cuff deflation.
- Active foot dorsiflexion and relaxation.

- The Valsalva maneuver. This may be the preferred technique to demonstrate saphenofemoral incompetence.[19]

Venous reflux is elicited by imaging the vein under investigation while applying compression to the extremity using one of the methods described. The compression is abruptly removed and the presence and duration of reflux observed (▶ Fig. 4.8). Pneumatic cuff deflation has been used to permit quantitative assessment of reflux. This may be the most reproducible, although some find it technically more difficult.

The patient is examined in a room with sufficient lighting to enable thorough evaluation of the lower extremities and establish the distribution of varices.

The lower extremities are inspected for varicosities and scars from surgery to help predict the source of reflux and facilitate the examination.

Reflux is more likely to develop later in the day, especially for nondilated vein segments. A warm environment helps to make veins dilate, while a cold environment can cause them to constrict, making them difficult to see so that borderline venous reflux may disappear. The lower extremity under investigation must be relaxed during imaging to allow good venous filling in the calf veins.

4.4.2 Suggested Protocols for Scanning the Great Saphenous Vein, Deep Veins above Knee, and Thigh Perforators

The patient should stand facing toward the examiner with the leg rotated outward, heel on the ground, and weight taken on the opposite extremity (▶ Fig. 4.6).

Start the scan in the groin of the first extremity to be examined. Use a transverse view to identify the GSV and the CFV, both lying medial to the common femoral artery (▶ Fig. 4.3). Several veins can be visualized in the region of the SFJ, and two GSV valves (terminal and preterminal) can be imaged near the SFJ. It is important to assess these tributaries and GSV valves as several hemodynamic patterns can be seen.

Evaluate possible sources of reflux or proximal points of insufficiency including SFJ incompetence (▶ Fig. 4.9), veins from the lower abdomen or pelvis, thigh or calf perforators, or the vein of Giacomini. If there are changes in competence, note the distance from landmarks such as the groin or knee crease.

In the transverse view, determine whether the destination for reflux is into (1) the GSV within the

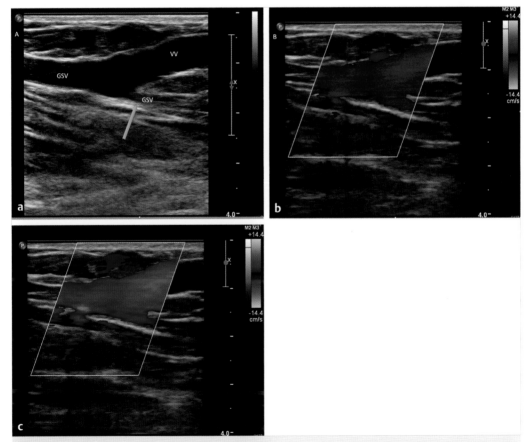

Fig. 4.9 Saphenofemoral junction incompetence with significant venous reflux in the proximal great saphenous vein (GSV). **(a)** The proximal GSV feeds a superficial varicosity (VV) and becomes smaller in diameter distally (arrow). **(b)** During augmentation with color Doppler, antegrade blood flow is noted in blue. **(c)** Venous reflux noted in red after augmentation.

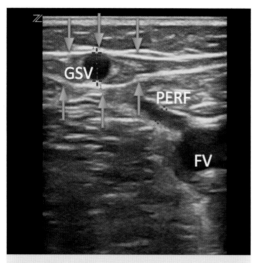

Fig. 4.10 The saphenous compartment: B-mode ultrasound showing the left great saphenous vein (GSV) in the saphenous compartment (arrows) at the level of the midthigh. Of note, there is a perforating vein (PERF) that communicates with the femoral vein (FV) at that level.

saphenous compartment, (2) the accessory anterior saphenous vein which is slightly external to GSV and aligned with the femoral vessels below, or (3) major thigh tributaries superficial to the saphenous fascia.

Follow the full length of the GSV or tributaries to the ankle. This vein lies within a fascial compartment, which can easily be identified on the B-mode ultrasound image (▶ Fig. 4.10). Test every few centimeters for compressibility and reflux.

Measure diameters at the junction and along the GSV if there is reflux. Suggested sites of measurements are 3 to 5 cm below the SFJ, at the midthigh, and at the knee.[4,20] The measurement should be made of the saphenous trunk vein and not of any varix or dilated segment with an incompetent valve. Measurement of the diameter can be used to help decide between different types of treatment, such as sclerotherapy, radiofrequency or endovenous laser ablation, and surgery.[4] The depth of the saphenous trunk beneath the skin is also important in patients being considered for endovenous thermal therapy.[21] These measurements can be used as a baseline for follow-up after endovenous procedures.

The CFV should be tested in the longitudinal view for phasic flow with normal respiration, cessation of flow with deep inspiration, possible reflux with the Valsalva maneuver, and flow during manual compression of the thigh or calf (▶ Fig. 4.11). This may be better demonstrated with the patient in the supine position. If continuous flow is detected in the CFV (loss of phasicity), which can indicate a proximal obstruction, it is recommended to extend duplex scanning to the iliac veins and inferior vena cava.

The CFV should be examined above and below the SFJ as retrograde flow in the CFV is seen at the SFJ level or higher in the presence of SFJ reflux, whereas retrograde flow distal to this level represents true deep venous reflux. It is then necessary to follow the full length of the FV to the POPV. The external iliac vein may not have a single valve, so it need not be checked for incompetence.[17]

It is recommended to look for perforators on the medial aspect of the thigh during the examination of the GSV and the deep veins (▶ Fig. 4.10). Not all thigh perforators, competent or incompetent, will be detected. These are usually found in the middle and lower thirds of the thigh, but can also occur in the proximal thigh near the SFJ. It is necessary to look for lateral and posterior thigh perforators if clinical assessment shows varices in these regions.

Use spectral and/or color Doppler to test for inward and outward flow in perforators by calf or thigh muscle contraction. Perforating veins that allow bidirectional flow are probably abnormal, although a few nonvaricose patients may have a similar pattern. If an incompetent thigh perforating vein is found, then it may be useful to record its diameter measured at the muscle fascia and its location with reference to the knee joint to help decide the best management for this vein.

4.4.3 Suggested Protocols for Scanning the Popliteal Vein

The popliteal fossa is a difficult site for investigation, showing a complex anatomy and different patterns of venous flow. Multiple longitudinal and transverse views are required. POPV is properly scanned with the patient lying in prone position. The POPV should be examined above and below the SPJ when this is present given that retrograde POPV flow is present above the SPJ when the SPJ terminal valve is incompetent, and only retrograde flow distal to this level represents true deep venous reflux. The anatomic and hemodynamic relationship of the POPV, SPJ, and gastrocnemius veins should be established.

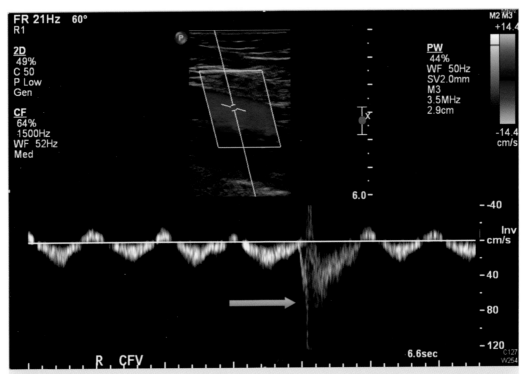

Fig. 4.11 Doppler ultrasound evaluation of the common femoral vein (CFV). Spectral waveforms show normal phasicity and augmentation (arrow).

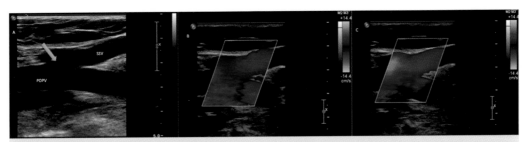

Fig. 4.12 (a) Longitudinal ultrasound image at the level of the saphenopopliteal junction (arrow). **(b)** During augmentation with Color Doppler, antegrade blood flow is noted in blue. **(c)** Venous reflux noted in red after augmentation.

4.4.4 Suggested Protocols for Scanning the SSV, Thigh Extension of the SSV, and Vein of Giacomini

Scan the SSV, thigh extension of SSV, and vein of Giacomini with the patient standing and facing away, with the knee slightly bent, heel on the ground, and weight taken on the opposite extremity.

Start at the back of the knee. Use a transverse view to identify the major veins of the popliteal fossa. Determine whether the SPJ is present. If so, show the junction in a longitudinal view (▸ Fig. 4.4). Test the POPV proximal and distal to the SPJ, the gastrocnemius vein insertion, and the SPJ for reflux or thrombosis. Determine if there is SPJ incompetence with SSV reflux (▸ Fig. 4.12). If there are changes in competence, note the distance from landmarks such as the malleoli or knee crease. SSV reflux may occur during calf muscle contraction or manual calf compression (systolic phase) in some patients, suggesting possible popliteal and/or FV obstruction, whereas typically reflux is most obvious during calf release (diastolic phase). If there is reflux, measure the diameter of the SSV 3 cm distal to the SPJ (or at the popliteal crease) and at midcalf, avoiding any varix in the vein. Measure the level of the SPJ in relation to the popliteal skin crease. The SSV may join the POPV medially, posteriorly, or laterally, so it is advisable to record its position in relation to the POPV circumference. Ascertain the presence or absence of an artery accompanying the SSV or the gastrocnemius veins. This is of importance when ultrasound-guided sclerotherapy is to be considered. The sural nerve runs parallel to the SSV from midcalf down to the heel. If the SSV is incompetent, make note in the report if the sural nerve is in intimate contact with the vein. They can be confused during surgery or the nerve may be damaged during interventional procedures such as endovenous thermal ablation.[22] Look for alternative sources of reflux including communication of the SSV with a popliteal fossa perforator, GSV tributaries, pelvic veins traced to the buttock or perineum, the thigh extension of SSV, or the vein of Giacomini. Look for alternative destinations for GSV reflux including tributaries, the thigh extension of SSV, or the vein of Giacomini.

Scan the thigh extension of the SSV and its connections with deep thigh veins or pelvic veins. Determine its distal SSV connection and proximal connection into the GSV. Demonstrate the flow direction and show whether there is reflux down from saphenofemoral incompetence to pass to the SSV or up from saphenopopliteal incompetence to pass to the GSV.[23]

4.4.5 Suggested Protocols for Scanning Veins below the Knee

Scan for below-knee veins with the patient standing (preferable for superficial veins), or sitting with the foot hanging down resting on the examiner's knee or on a step.

With experience, all deep crural veins can be identified. Examine PTVs from a medial or posteromedial view and PerVs from a posteromedial or posterior view.

These veins should be examined in patients with past or present deep vein thrombosis (DVT), and in patients with incompetent perforating veins in the calf. PerVs are the most frequently affected calf veins following previous venous thrombosis.[24] Examination of soleal and gastrocnemius veins deep in their muscle groups completes the basic investigation of deep veins in the lower extremity.

Examine the GSV in the calf for venous reflux. Following varicose vein surgery, incompetence of the GSV below the knee may fill varices at the ankle and in the foot. Examine the posterior arch vein, which is a major tributary of the GSV in the leg, search for calf perforating veins that join this vein in the medial calf region, and test for reflux in the vein that may result in medial calf varices.[25]

Examination of Calf Perforators

Perforators pass through the deep fascia, which is a distinct band on the B-mode image (▶ Fig. 4.13). Look for perforators around the circumference of the calf. Flow direction should always be

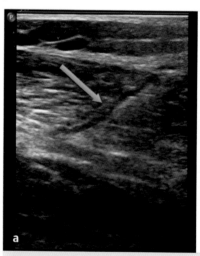
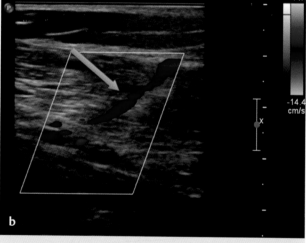

Fig. 4.13 Ultrasound images showing a perforating vein (arrow) at the level of the calf. **(a)** B-mode ultrasound and **(b)** color Doppler showing antegrade blood flow from the superficial to the deep venous systems.

superficial to deep (competent). Not all calf perforators, competent or incompetent, will be detected. If they show outward flow, then measure their diameters at the deep fascia and their level from the medial or lateral malleolus. However, diameter measurement alone cannot distinguish competent from incompetent perforators. Test for bidirectional flow by color Doppler or spectral analysis after a distal muscle squeeze or isometric calf muscle contraction. However, no consensus has been reached on the pathologic significance of bidirectional flow. Bidirectional flow in a perforator indicates its incompetence, but some authors argue that true pathologic incompetence is present only if reflux is elicited during the diastolic phase of calf muscle relaxation or release of compression.[26] Any incompetent perforating veins or competent perforators with diameters above 3 mm should be noted in the report.

Deep venous incompetence or current DVT is important to exclude as a cause for the patient's symptoms. Postthrombotic syndrome in patients with a past history of DVT can lead to deep venous incompetence.

Common perforators: The most common perforating veins are shown in ▶ Fig. 1.8. Cockett's perforators are by far the most common. These are medial, paratibial in the distal two-thirds of the lower leg.

4.5 Documentation and Reporting Nomenclature

Reporting should be in accordance with the American College of Radiology (ACR)–AIUM–SRU practice guideline for the performance of peripheral venous ultrasound examination, ACR–SPR–SRU practice guideline for performing and interpreting diagnostic ultrasound examinations, and ACR practice guideline for communication of diagnostic imaging findings.[27]

Adequate documentation is essential for high-quality patient care. There should be a permanent record of the ultrasound examination and its interpretation. Comparison with prior relevant imaging studies may prove helpful. Images of all appropriate areas, both normal and abnormal, should be recorded. Variations from normal size should generally be accompanied by measurements. Images should be labeled with the patient identification, facility identification, examination date, and image orientation. The report should state the reason for undertaking the investigation. An official interpretation (final report) of the ultrasound examination

should be included in the patient's medical record. Retention of the ultrasound examination images should be consistent both with clinical need and with relevant legal and local health care facility requirements.

The emphasis of an investigation for the morphology and hemodynamic changes in patients with chronic venous disease in the lower extremities (Duplex US mapping) is quite different from a test for suspected DVT. The request for the investigation should be made by a physician who has taken a history and undertaken clinical examination to provide valid reasons for the investigation and guidance as to what to look for.

A Duplex US study should include the following minimum images:
- CFV bifurcation.
- FV proximal and distal demonstrating patency and competency.
- POPV demonstrating patency and competency.
- SFJ demonstrating patency and competency.
- SPJ (if present) demonstrating patency and competency.
- Any incompetent perforators noting their diameter, depth, and position relative to a surface landmark.
- Any significant or atypical junctions of varices to the normal system.
- Any incidental findings such as thrombus, Baker's cyst, or popliteal aneurysm:
  - Diagrammatic representation as well as a textual report is most helpful to express the findings. Video recordings can be useful for quality control purposes but would not normally be part of the report of the investigation.

Reports should detail information regarding venous reflux and development of varices or other aspects of venous disease. This should include the presence of incompetence at each saphenous junction and extent of reflux in each saphenous trunk, describing the GSV in the thigh and calf separately where appropriate. The morphology and hemodynamic abnormalities relating to varices and location of diseased veins should be indicated on a diagram. In cases of recurrent varices, it is useful to know whether recurrence has occurred at a previously ligated junction or whether a previously treated saphenous trunk has recanalized. Inclusion of the diameters of diseased veins including saphenous trunks and perforating veins is useful because this may influence the treatment selected for that vein. The report should also include information regarding the morphology of the veins that are hypoplastic or atretic or that have been removed at a previous operation.

Deep or superficial veins that have suffered recent or previous venous thrombosis should be described, including the current patency of the vein, indicating whether the vein remained occluded or has recanalized and whether the recanalized vein has become incompetent and to what extent.

The report should convey the full information obtained by the investigator to the physicians responsible for the patient's treatment. This should greatly influence the management of the patient, so the report should be as unambiguous as possible. This informative process is obviously facilitated if the investigator and clinician responsible for treatment are the same person, but a comprehensive report with a diagram is always suggested for treatment and subsequent follow-up.

4.6 Quality Control and Improvement, Safety, Infection Control, Patient Education, and Training of Personnel Conducting Venous Duplex Ultrasound Examinations

Policies and procedures related to quality, patient education, infection control, and safety should be developed and implemented in accordance with the ACR Policy on Quality Control and Improvement, Safety, Infection Control and Patient Education appearing under the heading Position Statement on QC & Improvement, Safety, Infection Control, and Patient Education on the ACR web site (http://www.acr.org/guidelines). Equipment performance monitoring should be in accordance with the ACR Technical Standard for Diagnostic Medical Physics Performance Monitoring of Real Time Ultrasound Equipment.

There is considerable variation between countries as to who actually undertakes the investigation. Registered vascular technologists usually perform these tests in the United States and Australia, vascular scientists in the United Kingdom, and radiologists in many other countries. However, it is common for surgeons, angiologists, and phlebologists to perform their own investigations. It is highly desirable that all personnel involved in performing the investigations undergo systematic training that should include theoretic information, practical training, and clinical experience of the investigation recorded in a logbook. Reliable information can only be obtained from duplex ultrasound examinations performed by staff who have a detailed knowledge of the pathologic conditions for which they are searching.

References

[1] Gloviczki P, Comerota AJ, Dalsing MC, et al. Society for Vascular Surgery, American Venous Forum. The care of patients with varicose veins and associated chronic venous diseases: clinical practice guidelines of the Society for Vascular Surgery and the American Venous Forum. J Vasc Surg. 2011; 53(5) Suppl:2S–48S

[2] Stonebridge PA, Chalmers N, Beggs I, Bradbury AW, Ruckley CV. Recurrent varicose veins: a varicographic analysis leading to a new practical classification. Br J Surg. 1995; 82(1):60–62

[3] Jutley RS, Cadle I, Cross KS. Preoperative assessment of primary varicose veins: a duplex study of venous incompetence. Eur J Vasc Endovasc Surg. 2001; 21(4):370–373

[4] Coleridge-Smith P, Labropoulos N, Partsch H, Myers K, Nicolaides A, Cavezzi A. Duplex ultrasound investigation of the veins in chronic venous disease of the lower limbs—UIP consensus document. Part I. Basic principles. Eur J Vasc Endovasc Surg. 2006; 31(1):83–92

[5] Kachlik D, Pechacek V, Musil V, Baca V. The deep venous system of the lower extremity: new nomenclature. Phlebology. 2012; 27(2):48–58

[6] Caggiati A, Bergan JJ, Gloviczki P, Jantet G, Wendell-Smith CP, Partsch H, International Interdisciplinary Consensus Committee on Venous Anatomical Terminology. Nomenclature of the veins of the lower limbs: an international interdisciplinary consensus statement. J Vasc Surg. 2002; 36(2):416–422

[7] Caggiati A, Bergan JJ, Gloviczki P, Eklof B, Allegra C, Partsch H, International Interdisciplinary Consensus Committee on Venous Anatomical Terminology. Nomenclature of the veins of the lower limb: extensions, refinements, and clinical application. J Vasc Surg. 2005; 41(4):719–724

[8] Kachlik D, Pechacek V, Baca V, Musil V. The superficial venous system of the lower extremity: new nomenclature. Phlebology. 2010; 25(3):113–123

[9] Bergan JJ, Bunke N. The Vein Book. Oxford: Oxford University Press; 2014

[10] Pittathankal AA, Adamson M, Pursell R, Richards T, Galland RB, Magee TR. Duplex-defined spatial anatomy of the saphenopopliteal junction. Phlebology. 2006; 21(1):45–47

[11] Malgor RD, Labropoulos N. Diagnosis of venous disease with duplex ultrasound. Phlebology. 2013; 28 Suppl 1:158–161

[12] Labropoulos N, Tiongson J, Pryor L, et al. Definition of venous reflux in lower-extremity veins. J Vasc Surg. 2003; 38 (4):793–798

[13] Somjen GM, Royle JP, Fell G, Roberts AK, Hoare MC, Tong Y. Venous reflux patterns in the popliteal fossa. J Cardiovasc Surg (Torino). 1992; 33(1):85–91

[14] Jiang P, van Rij AM, Christie R, Hill G, Solomon C, Thomson I. Recurrent varicose veins: patterns of reflux and clinical severity. Cardiovasc Surg. 1999; 7(3):332–339

[15] Fischer R, Linde N, Duff C, Jeanneret C, Chandler JG, Seeber P. Late recurrent saphenofemoral junction reflux after ligation and stripping of the greater saphenous vein. J Vasc Surg. 2001; 34(2):236–240

[16] Yamaki T, Nozaki M, Sasaki K. Color duplex-guided sclerotherapy for the treatment of venous malformations. Dermatol Surg. 2000; 26(4):323–328

[17] Khilnani NM, Grassi CJ, Kundu S, et al. Cardiovascular Interventional Radiological Society of Europe, American College of Phlebology, and Society of Interventional Radiology Standards of Practice Committees. Multi-society consensus quality improvement guidelines for the treatment of lower-extremity superficial venous insufficiency with endovenous thermal ablation from the Society of Interventional Radiology, Cardiovascular Interventional Radiological Society of Europe, American College of Phlebology and Canadian Interventional Radiology Association. J Vasc Interv Radiol. 2010; 21(1):14–31

[18] Kundu S, Grassi CJ, Khilnani NM, et al. Cardiovascular Interventional Radiological Society of Europe, American College of Phlebology, and Society of Interventional Radiology Standards of Practice Committees. Multi-disciplinary quality improvement guidelines for the treatment of lower extremity superficial venous insufficiency with ambulatory phlebectomy from the Society of Interventional Radiology, Cardiovascular Interventional Radiological Society of Europe, American College of Phlebology and Canadian Interventional Radiology Association. J Vasc Interv Radiol. 2010; 21(1):1–13

[19] Baker SR, Burnand KG, Sommerville KM, Thomas ML, Wilson NM, Browse NL. Comparison of venous reflux assessed by duplex scanning and descending phlebography in chronic venous disease. Lancet. 1993; 341(8842):400–403

[20] Joh JH, Park H-C. The cutoff value of saphenous vein diameter to predict reflux. J Korean Surg Soc. 2013; 85(4):169–174

[21] Sichlau MJ, Ryu RK. Cutaneous thermal injury after endovenous laser ablation of the great saphenous vein. J Vasc Interv Radiol. 2004; 15(8):865–867

[22] Kerver ALA, van der Ham AC, Theeuwes HP, et al. The surgical anatomy of the small saphenous vein and adjacent nerves in relation to endovenous thermal ablation. J Vasc Surg. 2012; 56(1):181–188

[23] Delis KT, Knaggs AL, Khodabakhsh P. Prevalence, anatomic patterns, valvular competence, and clinical significance of the Giacomini vein. J Vasc Surg. 2004; 40(6):1174–1183

[24] Labropoulos N, Webb KM, Kang SS, et al. Patterns and distribution of isolated calf deep vein thrombosis. J Vasc Surg. 1999; 30(5):787–791

[25] Meissner MH. Lower extremity venous anatomy. Semin Intervent Radiol. 2005; 22(3):147–156

[26] Cappelli M, Ermini S, Turchi A, Bono G. Considérations hemodynamiques sur les perforantes. Phlebologie. 1958; 47 (4):389–393

[27] American Institute of Ultrasound in Medicine, American College of Radiology, Society of Radiologists in Ultrasound. Practice guideline for the performance of peripheral venous ultrasound examinations. J Ultrasound Med. 2011; 30 (1):143–150

5 Compression Therapy

Erica A. Gupta, Raphael J. Yoo, Carlos Alberto M. Carvalho, and Felipe B. Collares

5.1 Introduction

Compression therapy has been used for thousands of years in the practical treatment of wounds and ulcers, with the earliest documentation of compression bandages dating back to the Neolithic Age (5,000–2,500 BC).[1] Throughout the more recent centuries, physicians and surgeons have employed compression therapy for the treatment of wounds/ulcers, primarily using inelastic material such as plaster bandages/dressings. Elastic compression bandages were developed in the mid-1800s after Charles Goodyear developed a process by which to increase the durability and elasticity of rubber. In 1885, German dermatologist Dr. Paul Unna developed an elastic bandage impregnated with zinc oxide paste to help promote healing, which currently is known as the "Unna's boot."

In modern medical practice, compression therapy continues to demonstrate an important role in prevention and therapy for a variety of venous diseases, for example, perioperative venous thrombosis, varicose veins, postthrombotic syndrome (PTS), and venous stasis ulcers. There are hundreds of products available on the market today that offer varying degrees of compression. It is imperative that the prescribing provider has an understanding of the pathophysiology of venous disease to guide clinical management, and is also familiar with different products and their specific intended uses.

5.2 Mechanism of Action

The goal of compression therapy is to counteract the effects of gravity upon the venolymphatic circulation. Namely, pressure exerted on an area of the body's surface with elastic or inelastic materials will help to decrease ambulatory venous hypertension and interstitial pressures to prevent malfunction resulting in venous and lymphatic disorders.[1]

5.2.1 Laplace's Law

Laplace's law in relation to compression states that external pressure (P) is directly proportional to the tension of material (T) and inversely proportional to the radius of curvature (R) to which tension is applied ($P = T/R$).[2,3] Applied to the use of compression bandages/stockings, the law of Laplace dictates that the greatest amount of external pressure will be directed to the ankle (~100%), and external pressure progressively decreases as the radius of the leg increases more proximally (~70% at the knee, ~ 40% at the thigh). This provides the basis for the decreasing graduated compression concept (► Fig. 5.1).

5.2.2 Physiology Consequences of Compression

The pressure exerted by compression on the surface of the skin is transmitted to the level of both the superficial and deep blood vessels, helping to improve local venolymphatic circulation at multiple levels.

Edema

By applying external compression, the pressure on the tissues works to counteract filtration, preventing reflux of fluid as well as promoting resorption

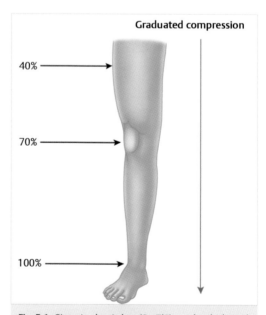

Fig. 5.1 Given Laplace's law ($P = T/R$), as the thickness/radius of the leg decreases toward the ankle, greater pressure will be exerted.

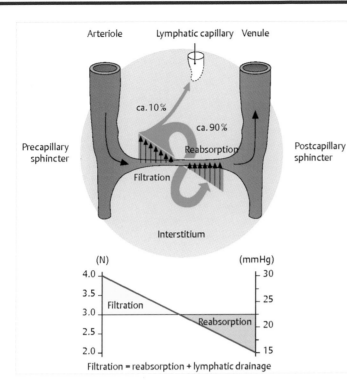

Fig. 5.2 The normal mechanism of lymphatic filtration and reabsorption. (Used with permission from Schuenke M, Schulte E, Schumacher U. General Anatomy and Musculoskeletal System. Stuttgart: Thieme; 2010. Illustration by Karl Wesker.)

of excess fluid from the interstitial space (▶ Fig. 5.2, ▶ Fig. 5.3). Compression stockings have been shown to decrease limb volume and pain associated with limb edema.[4,5,6,7]

Lymphatic Circulation

Compression combined with movement or exercise has been shown to improve contraction of the lymphatic system.[8,9] Even more important is the impact that compression has upon the capillary bed and downstream lymphatic circulation. Applied compression results in closer proximity of the skin and subcutaneous tissues to the superficial capillary network. This contact results in improved capillary resorption as well as restricted capillary filtration, reducing the lymphatic load (▶ Fig. 5.2, ▶ Fig. 5.3). Because compression results in disproportionate removal of water compared to proteins from the tissues, the tissue oncotic pressure increases. This phenomenon necessitates ongoing compression therapy to prevent reaccumulation of water in the tissues, which is important in cases of chronic edema where success is dependent on continued compression. Compression is also shown to have an effect on the breakdown of fibrosclerotic tissue and downregulation of proinflammatory cytokines, reducing membrane permeability and leakage.[10]

Venous Circulation

Compression affects the venous circulation by transmitting pressure to narrow or even occlude the superficial and deep venous vessels. The amount of external pressure required to diminish the venous diameter is dependent on body positioning. When a patient is recumbent, pressures as low as 10 to 15 mm Hg are sufficient to reduce venous diameter.[11] Pressures of 20 to 25 mm Hg are sufficient in compressing the superficial veins in the supine position, while pressures of 35 to 40 mm Hg are required in the upright position.[12,13] Other studies have shown that when using an external blood pressure cuff inflated to 40 to 60 mm Hg in patients with known incompetent valves, they were able to have noticeable decrease or complete resolution of venous reflux as well as decrease in vein diameter.[14,15] This phenomena was also noted in patients with congenital absence of venous valves, indicating that improvement in reflux and ambulatory venous hypertension may in part be related to the degree of resistance to retrograde flow provided by external compression and not just related to improved valve closure.[16]

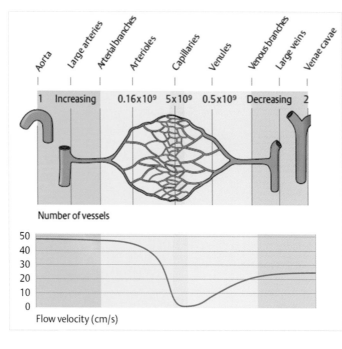

Fig. 5.3 Normal flow velocity across the capillary bed. (Used with permission from Schuenke M, Schulte E, Schumacher U. General Anatomy and Musculoskeletal System. Stuttgart: Thieme; 2010. Illustration by Karl Wesker.)

Capillary Circulation

By increasing local tissue pressure, compression accelerates blood flow in capillaries and reduces capillary filtration, resulting in improved venous flow, improved distribution of microcirculation blood flow, and normalization of leukocyte adhesion (▶ Fig. 5.2, ▶ Fig. 5.3).[17,18,19,20,21,22,23] Compression therapy also contributes to ulcer healing by increasing flow volume, thereby reducing endothelial interaction with leukocytes and activation of the inflammatory cascade, which can lead to increased membrane permeability and microvascular damage.[24] Compression also has an indirect mechanical effect in venous leg ulcers by tightening the intracellular junctions between endothelial cells, which has a role in reducing proinflammatory cytokines.[25,26]

Arterial Circulation

The impact of compression therapy on arterial circulation is also important in consideration of compression therapy. With the degree of external compression applied comes the risk of reduction of not only venous diameter but also arterial diameter. It is suggested that pressures above 60 mm Hg will decrease local arterial perfusion, particularly in the recumbent patient. Studies have shown that skin necrosis and ulceration have occurred during prolonged compression, possibly related to unrecognized/occult peripheral arterial occlusive disease.[27] For patients with critical limb ischemia (ankle-brachial index [ABI] < 0.5), sustained compression therapy is therefore a contraindication. However, it is now felt that patients with systolic ankle pressures between 60 and 100 mm Hg in the supine position may still benefit from inelastic compression, using 40 mm Hg or less as an initial pressure with the basis that the massaging effect of compression during ambulation will help to increase venous return and improve the arteriovenous pressure gradient, resulting in improved arterial flow.[28]

5.3 Types of Compression Therapy

Compression therapy includes many different devices made of various materials, including graduated compression stockings, bandages, boots, and intermittent pneumatic compression devices. Therapies are generally divided into elastic and inelastic techniques based upon the extensibility (or stretch) of the material with which the device is made.

5.3.1 Inelastic Compression

Inelastic devices include short stretch and no stretch (i.e., inextensible) options, which include the gauze boots (Unna's boot), dressings, pneumatic compression devices, and inelastic bandages and garments. Inelastic bandages produce high "working pressures" during ambulation and lower "resting pressures." Because extensibility is dependent on the contraction of muscle, there is little variation in the pressure exerted on the superficial vessels. Furthermore, if the muscle pump is ineffective (as in patients with muscle atrophy or immobility), then the benefit of inelastic compression is limited.[1,29,30]

The most well-known inelastic compression device is the Unna's boot, which is composed of a colorless gelatin crepe bandage impregnated with glycerin and zinc oxide paste.[31] The Unna's boot is used in the treatment of ulcers resulting from chronic venous insufficiency because it results in local pressure when the patient ambulates while simultaneously promoting ulcer healing. Because it requires several days of use to exert maximal effectiveness, care must be taken so that pressure is not excessive enough to cause limb ischemia. Therefore, it is imperative that an experienced team directs application and management of the Unna's boot.

Pneumatic compression devices are another well-known inelastic device commonly used for deep vein thrombosis (DVT) prevention and also applied primarily at night for patients with refractory edema and venous ulcers.

5.3.2 Elastic Compression

Elastic compression consists of extensible or long-stretch materials, such as compression stockings, multilayer elastic wraps, and elastic bandages. Elastic compression works in all positions, including the supine position. Unlike inelastic compression, elastic compression must be removed at night to avoid arterial inflow problems.[32]

Compression Stockings

Elastic compression stockings have both short- and long-term applications. Common applications for short-term therapy include in the postsurgical setting as well as following endovenous therapies and sclerotherapy. Long-term use may be indicated in patients with chronic venous insufficiency. Compression stockings should be routinely adjusted as the diameter of the leg and edema decrease/stabilize to ensure a proper fit.

Compression Stocking/Bandage Pressures

The sub-bandage pressure is determined by a combination of three things: material stiffness and elasticity, size and shape of the leg, and activity level of the patient.[33] The universally adopted unit of measure for pressure exerted by elastic compression stockings is millimeters of mercury (mm Hg), which has been the measure used worldwide in studies regarding compression therapy.[3,34]

Style and Sizing

It is important that clinicians have the necessary training and adhere to guidelines for assessing and caring for patients who wear compression stockings.[33] Wearing an improperly fitted stocking can result in pressure-induced necrosis related to inadequate perfusion. In cases where the stocking is too long, the stocking may roll down and effectively create a tourniquet for the remaining lower extremity. Therefore, the amount of lengthwise stretch is also an important factor to consider to prevent stockings from slipping down.[32]

Elastic stockings come in various different lengths. The particular style and length for a patient is best determined by the type and degree of disease, but other factors to consider are ease of use, comfort, and cost. Compression stockings can be custom made or standard fit.

- *Knee-high stockings* end just below the knee. While they do not treat pathology in the thigh, they will help to prevent accumulation of fluid in the lower leg and sequelae of chronic edema, venous insufficiency, and varicose veins. This style tends to be best tolerated by the patient and is also the easiest to apply and least expensive.
- *Thigh-high stockings* extend to the upper/mid-thigh level. These can be useful in patients who have significant pathology in the thigh or who have undergone vein ablative therapy/surgery to the level of the thigh to prevent recanalization (▶ Fig. 5.4).
- *Full-length stockings* or tights include coverage from the foot to the level of the hips. Full-length stockings can cover one leg or both legs. For patients who feel that the stocking is too oppressive, some brands can be ordered with the foot open to air.

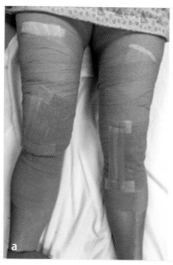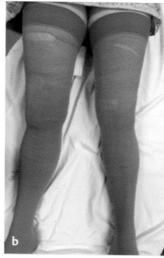

Fig. 5.4 Pressure dressings (left) followed by application of thigh-high compression stockings (right) in a patient post sclerotherapy.

Compression stocking sizes and fits vary by manufacturer, so it is important to obtain accurate measurements prior to prescribing the stockings. Once measurements are obtained, the stockings can be appropriately fitted for maximum comfort and benefit, which will help to improve patient compliance.

Materials

Compression stockings can be made from a variety of materials, including nylon, cotton, spandex, and natural rubber. The most commonly used material in elastic stockings is spandex with different proportions of added cotton or other materials.[3] The combination and thickness of the fibers determines the elasticity of the stocking.

Use of Stockings

Stockings that are to be worn every day should be prescribed for a period of 3 to 6 months and should be replaced with new stockings after the recommended time period.[28,29] It is important that before the stockings are replaced, the patient is reevaluated by a physician to determine whether the pressure gradient needs to be adjusted or can be maintained. Stockings generally should be put on in the morning and taken off at night to sleep; however, their use should be individualized.[35] When the stocking is too tight at the calf, it can cause a feeling of strangulation, and is an incorrect fit for that patient. An important factor to improve the clinical course of the venous disease is the daily use of stockings. However, due to a variety of reasons, which can include patient discomfort as well as technical difficulty in use, many patients end up not using the stockings as recommended by their physician.[36] A systematic review of compression hosiery found that patients who complied with wearing stockings tended to be older or had endured their symptoms longer.[33] Patients may be noncompliant with wearing stockings if they feel they do not work or they are too tight or too hot.[33] In addition, patients who are obese or elderly may have difficulty applying the stockings, leading to noncompliance.[13]

5.4 Clinical Indications

For many years, compression therapy was based on empiric studies. However, with more recent prospective and detailed randomized studies by different medical societies and with the rise of dedicated research by various authors, the International Compression Club was created where parameters were established for the use of graduated compression pressures in stockings.[30]

5.4.1 Prevention of Varicose Veins and Telangiectasias

The etiology of varicose veins has not yet been fully elucidated. Data suggest that a molecular defect in the vessel wall leads to dilation of the vein, and anatomic abnormalities result in disturbances of hemodynamics that promote progression of disease. Because the deep venous system is encased by a musculofibrous sheath, these veins can accommodate changes in blood pressure that increase the volume of the vessel. Conversely, the superficial veins are not contained within a sheath and valves become incompetent when the vessel lumen expands beyond capacity. Blood is then routed into smaller vessels and produces abnormal dilation, resulting in clinically visible varicose veins and telengiactasias.[11]

External compression of previously untreated veins by bandages or graduated stockings produces pressure to move blood toward the heart rather than outward to the vessel wall. There are no randomized controlled trials demonstrating that compression therapy prevents progression of venous disease. However, patients with varicose veins report relief of symptoms with all classes of compression stockings.[37,38,39] Physiologic improvement in varicose veins only occurs with 30 to 50 mm Hg stockings.[11]

The need for compression therapy prior to an intervention remains highly controversial. Ablation of varicosities has proven more efficacious and cost-effective in the treatment of superficial reflux and argues against a trial of compression therapy prior to ablation as required by many third-party payers.[13]

5.4.2 Sclerotherapy

Sclerotherapy involves injection of a liquid or foam sclerosing agent into the targeted vessels causing inflammation and focal thrombosis of the target vessel, eventually resulting in permanent obliteration and fibrosis. Sclerotherapy is one of many minimally invasive treatment options available for the treatment of varicose veins and has been found to be safe. Sclerotherapy has demonstrated decreased wound infection and neovascularization compared to conventional surgery, with significant improvement in clinical and quality-of-life metrics.[40]

Compression therapy serves several purposes following sclerotherapy of varicose veins, including direct apposition of the treated vein walls to produce better fibrosis, decreased thrombus formation and subsequent risk of recanalization and postsclerosis pigmentation, prevention of telangiectatic matting, improvement of the physiologic function of the calf muscle pump, and increased blood flow through the deep venous system which prevents damage to the valves by the sclerosing agent.[11]

One study found that patients who used postsclerotherapy elastic compression stockings had a statistically significant degree of symptom improvement at 6 weeks compared to those who did not use compression stockings.[41] In addition,

patients who wore the compression stockings for 3 weeks had less postsclerotherapy hyperpigmentation compared with those who wore them for a shorter duration. Finally, there was less bruising, telangiectatic matting, edema, and ulceration in those who wore compression stockings compared to those who did not wear stockings.[41]

Stockings in the 20 to 30 mm Hg pressure range at the ankle have beneficial effects after sclerotherapy of small telangiectasias. However, a compression pressure of 30 to 40 mm Hg at the ankle corresponds to approximately 10 to 20 mm Hg elsewhere in the leg and is generally recommended for better outcomes.[42] Some physicians support the use of foam pads or rolled cotton wool to augment local pressure beneath the compression stocking (▶ Fig. 5.5).

Histologic studies have demonstrated that fibrous occlusion of a vessel generally requires at least 6 weeks following sclerotherapy, which supports continuous compression stocking use during the postoperative course. However, studies have shown that results were maintained in the long term whether compression therapy was used for 3 weeks or 6 weeks following sclerotherapy.[43]

The use of compression following sclerotherapy of telangiectasias has not been uniformly adopted. However, a multicenter study of the bilateral legs compared the use of a 30 to 40 mm Hg stocking over a cotton ball dressing for 3 days to a cotton ball dressing alone for 2 hours. Legs in the compression group demonstrated better outcomes for veins in the distal leg or for vessels greater than 0.5 mm in diameter.[42]

5.4.3 Endovenous Procedures

Endovenous laser ablation (EVLA) or radiofrequency ablation (RFA) therapies are minimally invasive therapies which involve thermal ablation of a targeted vessel. Thermal energy is targeted to generate occlusion and fibrosis of the targeted vessel. EVLA and RFA have been shown to have equal efficacy compared to that of conventional surgery, while maintaining decreased rates of wound infection and neovascularization and resulting in improved clinical and quality-of-life outcomes.[40]

Compression therapy has become the standard of care in patients undergoing EVLA or RFA. A recently published study suggested that the use of compression stockings for at least 7 days following endovenous laser therapy led to decreased pain and physical dysfunction compared to patients who only used stockings for 2 days.[44]

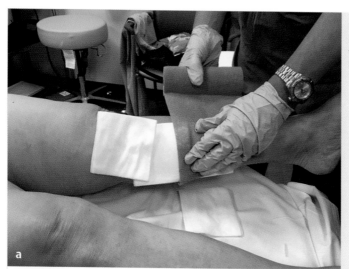

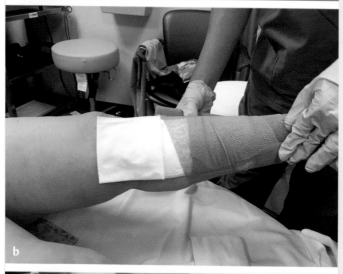

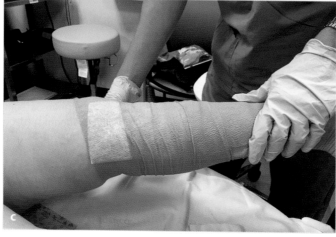

Fig. 5.5 Pads used with compression bandage to create more pressure over the desired area in the lower extremity.

Compression therapy is also routinely used after varicose vein surgery and has been shown to prevent superficial thrombophlebitis and DVT, improve wound healing, and reduce pain, bruising, and hematoma formation. Early ambulation is improved and return to work accelerated with the use of compression therapy following surgery.[11] It is important to use stockings with higher compression after varicose vein surgery, because they are more effective than lower compression. Although some authors recommend higher pressures (40–50 mm Hg),[45] most clinicians use stockings ranging from 30 to 40 mm Hg, as recommended by the Society for Vascular Surgery and American Venous Forum.[13] Finally, long-term compression may decrease recurrent varicosities and slow the progression of disease.

5.4.4 Edema and Venous Ulcers

Compression therapy is the most effective way to prevent or delay skin lesions that occur in chronic venous disease, and its efficacy has been proven in several randomized clinical trials.[46,47,48,49] Various types of compression and compression strengths have been studied, and on comparison of local therapy versus compression therapy, compression was found to promote faster healing in venous ulcers than local therapy alone. Several studies show different results in regard to success with ulcer healing, with varying results related to variations in technique as well as degree of patient noncompliance, with particular increases in noncompliance rates with higher pressure stockings.[50,51,52]

Finally, compression therapy is a mainstay in the management of chronic lymphedema. Initial treatment with bandages and compression hosiery has been found to be more effective in reducing lymphedema than hosiery alone.[53,54] However, as discussed with the physiology of water removal and elevation of oncotic pressures, long-term continued use of compression hosiery is essential to prevent reaccumulation.

5.4.5 Deep Vein Thrombosis and Postthrombotic Syndrome

DVT is a common problem in modern medicine with long-standing consequences if left untreated or suboptimally treated. Of these, the most severe consequence is PTS. PTS is a result of chronic thrombosis with resultant damage to the venous valves resulting in valvular dysfunction, which can ultimately lead to chronic lower extremity edema, increased risk of infections, and venous stasis ulcers. Various scoring systems for determining presence and severity of PTS (such as the Villalta score) are nonspecific, resulting in difficulties diagnosing patients with PTS.[55] Previous studies have shown that compression therapy has a role in both prevention and treatment of DVT and resultant PTS.[55,56,57,58,59] Studies of pneumatic compression devices and compression stockings have shown that both modalities reduce the risk of DVT in bedridden patients. In particular, elastic compression has proven beneficial in the prevention of postsurgical DVT alone and in conjunction with pharmacologic therapies. Though not widely practiced, compression in the setting of acute DVT in mobile patients has also been shown to reduce pain and swelling and prevent thrombus growth.[57,59,60]

However, recently some questions arose regarding the benefits of compression therapy in the prevention of PTS. One meta-analysis found that several studies performed regarding PTS are limited to small sample sizes and varying definitions for PTS.[56] A second meta-analysis found that two controlled studies showed prevention of occurrence of PTS in patients, while others did not find a significant difference.[55] One of the studies mentioned in the meta-analysis reported no significant decrease in PTS among users of compression stockings compared to placebo stockings.[58] Another study mentioned in the meta-analysis found that there was a gender difference with males reporting less relief/prevention of recurrence of symptoms compared to females, which was attributed to more noncompliance in the male gender.[55]

5.4.6 Superficial Thrombophlebitis

Superficial thrombophlebitis is a thrombotic process characterized by clotting in the superficial veins and associated with inflammatory changes and/or infection. There are no randomized controlled trials investigating compression therapy for the treatment of superficial thrombophlebitis. However, some authors advocate for the use of compression therapy for this indication, particularly in the thigh.[11,61] The theory is that the effect of gravity on the veins without external support will increase venous congestion and swelling, leading to increased pain. In addition to analgesics

Table 5.1 Classes of graded compression and clinical indications

Class	Indications
Class I: 8 to 12 mm Hg	Heaviness, fatigue in the leg
Class II: 15 to 20 mm Hg	Tired, aching legs, minor swelling, minor varicose veins
Class III: 20 to 30 mm Hg	Prophylaxis and treatment of mild vascular insufficiency, mild varicosities without significant edema
Class IV: 30 to 40 mm Hg	Varicose veins, chronic venous insufficiency, peripheral edema, prophylaxis postsurgical stripping, postphlebitic syndrome, varices in pregnancy, postligation or stripping
Class V: 40 to 50 mm Hg	Severe Class IV + marked dependent edema, venous ulcerations
Class VI: 50 to 60 mm Hg	Severe Class V + severe postthrombotic syndrome, irreversible lymphedema

and anti-inflammatory agents, ambulation, and, in some cases, topical anticoagulation, counteracting venous congestion with elastic compression can decrease these symptoms.

5.4.7 Pregnancy

Pregnant women can also use specific stockings to improve venous return, prevent venous disease, and reduce the effects of gestational edema. Prolonged valvular incompetence can result in fibrosis of the valves and chronic reflux that tends to occur more commonly in multiparous women. The use of compression stockings may prevent permanent damage to the valves during pregnancy. It is generally recommended that pregnant women use a 10 to 30 mm Hg compression pantyhose. However, if they have a history of varicosities or are multiparous, stockings of higher pressure (30–40 mm Hg) are recommended.[11]

A summary of recommendations for the use of medical stockings according to their compression pressure, based on the literature, including publications of the International Compression Club, is provided in ▶ Table 5.1.[29,45,62]

5.5 Complications and Contraindications

The most important contraindication to compression therapy is the presence of arterial occlusive disease. This is of particular concern in patients with venous ulcer disease, who have been shown to have concurrent moderate (13.6%) or severe (2.2%) lower extremity arterial disease.[63] These patients are at increased risk of ulceration from arterial occlusion secondary to compression therapy. Overall, an ABI less than 0.5 is considered a contraindication to compression therapy. However, compression therapy can be used safely in patients with arterial occlusive disease and an ABI > 0.5 after careful evaluation of peripheral pulses and with lower pressure bandages or stockings.[11]

Other contraindications to the use of compression stockings include inflammatory processes and cutaneous infections of the leg (e.g., septic phlebitis), congestive heart failure, hypersensitivity or allergy to the material, diabetic microangiopathy, or concurrent gangrene.[3,64]

Appropriately fitted stockings should alleviate pain, but ill-fitting stockings may increase pain and it is therefore important to perform a thorough clinical exam and maintain ongoing clinical evaluation of the patient on follow-up visits. In the first 1 to 2 weeks of use (when there may be some expected discomfort), patients may be given analgesics or consider a staged approach to compression. Additional complications of compression include the following: calf muscle atrophy (related to decreased activity in the setting of compression); skin problems such as maceration/increased exudate, itching, and allergic reactions; and pressure-related symptoms, particularly in patients with arterial disease, altered limb shape or limb deformity, reduced sensation, chronic systemic steroid use, or a chronic disease such as rheumatoid arthritis which impairs mobility.[30]

5.6 Conclusion

Although the use of elastic stockings has been reported for centuries, there is still much research to be done about compression therapy. Ongoing research is aimed at identifying ideal timing for initiation and ideal duration of compression therapy as well as research involving materials and fabrics used in the manufacture of compression stockings which will be better tolerated by patients and result in improved patient compliance. Compression stockings, as part of venous disease therapy, must be prescribed by a physician who knows the degree of compression indicated for the specific pathology of each individual patient. While much remains to be researched, several studies have shown that compression therapy significantly improves the quality of life of patients and remains an important part of treatment in venous disease.

References

[1] Mariani F, ed. Compression: Consensus Document Based on Scientific Literature and Clinical Experience. Torino: Edizioni Minerva Medica; 2009

[2] Franzeck UK, Spiegel I, Fischer M, Börtzler C, Stahel HU, Bollinger A. Combined physical therapy for lymphedema evaluated by fluorescence microlymphography and lymph capillary pressure measurements. J Vasc Res. 1997; 34 (4):306–311

[3] Belczak CEQ. Compressão na Patologia Linfática. In: Thomaz JB, Belczak CEQ, eds. Tratado de Flebologia e Linfologia. Rio de Janeiro: Rubio; 2006:839–850

[4] Muller-Buhl U, Heim B, Fischbach U, et al. Effect of compression stockings on leg volume in patients with varicose veins. Phlebology. 1998; 13:102–106

[5] Hamdan A. Management of varicose veins and venous insufficiency. JAMA. 2012; 308(24):2612–2621

[6] Meissner MH, Gloviczki P, Bergan J, et al. Primary chronic venous disorders. J Vasc Surg. 2007; 46 Suppl S:54S–67S

[7] Ibegbuna V, Delis KT, Nicolaides AN, Aina O. Effect of elastic compression stockings on venous hemodynamics during walking. J Vasc Surg. 2003; 37(2):420–425

[8] Olszewski WL. Lymph pressure and flow in limbs. In: Olszewski WL, ed. Lymph Stasis: Pathophysiology, Diagnosis and Treatment. Boca Raton, FL: CRC Press; 1991

[9] Olszewski WL. Contractility patterns of human leg lymphatics in various stages of obstructive lymphedema. Ann N Y Acad Sci. 2008; 1131:110–118

[10] Földi E, Sauerwald A, Hennig B. Effect of complex decongestive physiotherapy on gene expression for the inflammatory response in peripheral lymphedema. Lymphology. 2000; 33 (1):19–23

[11] Partsch H. Use of compression therapy. In: Goldman MP, Guex J-J, Weiss RA, eds. Sclerotherapy: Treatment of Varicose and Telangiectatic Leg Veins. Edinburgh: Saunders-Elsevier; 2011:123–155

[12] Partsch B, Partsch H. Calf compression pressure required to achieve venous closure from supine to standing positions. J Vasc Surg. 2005; 42(4):734–738

[13] Gloviczki P, Comerota AJ, Dalsing MC, et al. Society for Vascular Surgery, American Venous Forum. The care of patients with varicose veins and associated chronic venous diseases: clinical practice guidelines of the Society for Vascular Surgery and the American Venous Forum. J Vasc Surg. 2011; 53(5) Suppl:2S–48S

[14] Sarin S, Scurr JH, Coleridge Smith PD. Mechanism of action of external compression on venous function. Br J Surg. 1992; 79 (6):499–502

[15] Partsch H, Menzinger G, Borst-Krafek B, Groiss E. Does thigh compression improve venous hemodynamics in chronic venous insufficiency? J Vasc Surg. 2002; 36(5):948–952

[16] Partsch B, Mayer W, Partsch H. Improvement of ambulatory venous hypertension by narrowing of the femoral vein in congenital absence of venous valves. Phlebology. 1992; 7:101–104

[17] Onorati D, Rossi GG, Idiazabal G. Effect of elastic stockings on edema related to chronic venous insufficiency. Videocapillaroscopic assessment [in French]. J Mal Vasc. 2003; 28 (1):21–23

[18] Klopp R, Schippel W, Niemer W. Compression therapy and microcirculation: vital microscope investigations in patients suffering from chronic venous insufficiency before and after compression therapy. Phlebology. 1996; 11:19–25

[19] Galler S, Klyscz T, Jung MF, et al. Clinical efficacy of compression therapy and its influence on cutaneous microcirculation. Phlebology. 1995; 10:907–909

[20] Belcaro G, Gaspari AL, Legnini M, Napolitano AM, Marelli C. Evaluation of the effects of elastic compression in patients with chronic venous hypertension by laser-Doppler flowmetry. Acta Chir Belg. 1988; 88(3):163–167

[21] Allegra C, Olivia E, Sarcinella R. Hemodynamic modifications induced by compression therapy in CVI evaluated by microlymphography. Phlebology. 1995; 11(1):1138–1149

[22] Abu-Own A, Shami SK, Chittenden SJ, Farrah J, Scurr JH, Smith PD. Microangiopathy of the skin and the effect of leg compression in patients with chronic venous insufficiency. J Vasc Surg. 1994; 19(6):1074–1083

[23] Abu-Own A, Scurr JH, Smith PD, et al. Effect of compression on the skin microcirculation in chronic venous insufficiency. Phlebology. 1995; 10(1):5–11

[24] Horakova MA, Mayer W, Partsch H. Paramètres microcirculatoires, prédiction de la tendance a la cicatrisation des ulcères de jambe. Phlebologie. 1996; 49:461

[25] Herouy Y, Kahle B, Idzko M, et al. Tight junctions and compression therapy in chronic venous insufficiency. Int J Mol Med. 2006; 18(1):215–219

[26] Beidler SK, Douillet CD, Berndt DF, Keagy BA, Rich PB, Marston WA. Inflammatory cytokine levels in chronic venous insufficiency ulcer tissue before and after compression therapy. J Vasc Surg. 2009; 49(4):1013–1020

[27] Callam MJ, Ruckley CV, Dale JJ, Harper DR. Hazards of compression treatment of the leg: an estimate from Scottish surgeons. Br Med J (Clin Res Ed). 1987; 295(6610):1382

[28] Flour M, Clark M, Partsch H, et al. Dogmas and controversies in compression therapy: report of an International Compression Club (ICC) meeting, Brussels, May 2011. Int Wound J. 2013; 10(5):516–526

[29] Partsch H, Flour M, Smith PC, International Compression Club. Indications for compression therapy in venous and lymphatic disease consensus based on experimental data and scientific evidence. Under the auspices of the IUP. Int Angiol. 2008; 27(3):193–219

[30] Wound International. Compression in venous leg ulcers. A WUWHS consensus document. 2008

[31] Belczak CE, de Godoy JM, Ramos RN, de Oliveira MA, Belczak SQ, Caffaro RA. Is the wearing of elastic stockings for half a day as effective as wearing them for the entire day? Br J Dermatol. 2010; 162(1):42–45

[32] Neumann HAM. Compression therapy: European regulatory affairs. Phlebology. 2000; 15:182–187

[33] Palfreyman SJ, Michaels JA. A systematic review of compression hosiery for uncomplicated varicose veins. Phlebology. 2009; 24 Suppl 1:13–33

[34] Partsch H, Mosti G, Uhl JF. Unexpected venous diameter reduction by compression stocking of deep, but not superficial veins. Veins Lymphatics. 2012; 1:3

[35] Italian College of Phlebology. Guidelines on compression therapy. Acta Phlebologica. 2001; 2:3–24

[36] Cataldo JL, de Godoy JM, de Barros N. The use of compression stockings for venous disorders in Brazil. Phlebology. 2012; 27 (1):33–37

[37] Weiss RA, Duffy D. Clinical benefits of lightweight compression: reduction of venous-related symptoms by ready-to-wear lightweight gradient compression hosiery. Dermatol Surg. 1999; 25(9):701–704

[38] Jones NA, Webb PJ, Rees RI, Kakkar VV. A physiological study of elastic compression stockings in venous disorders of the leg. Br J Surg. 1980; 67(8):569–572

[39] Benigni JP, Sadoun S, Allaert FA, Vin F. Comparative study of the effectiveness of class 1 compression stockings on the symptomatology of early chronic venous disease. Phlebologie. 2003; 56:117–125

[40] Biemans AA, Kockaert M, Akkersdijk GP, et al. Comparing endovenous laser ablation, foam sclerotherapy, and conventional surgery for great saphenous varicose veins. J Vasc Surg. 2013; 58(3):727–34.e1

[41] Sadick NS, Sorhaindo L. An evaluation of post-sclerotherapy laser compression and its efficacy in the treatment of leg telangiectasias. Phlebology. 2006; 21(4):191–194

[42] Goldman MP, Beaudoing D, Marley W, Lopez L, Butie A. Compression in the treatment of leg telangiectasia: a preliminary report. J Dermatol Surg Oncol. 1990; 16(4):322–325

[43] Batch AJG, Wickremesinghe SS, Gannon ME, Dormandy JA. Randomised trial of bandaging after sclerotherapy for varicose veins. BMJ. 1980; 281(6237):423

[44] Bakker NA, Schieven LW, Bruins RM, van den Berg M, Hissink RJ. Compression stockings after endovenous laser ablation of the great saphenous vein: a prospective randomized controlled trial. Eur J Vasc Endovasc Surg. 2013; 46(5):588–592

[45] Mosti G. Post-treatment compression: duration and techniques. Phlebology. 2013; 28 Suppl 1:21–24

[46] Fletcher A, Cullum N, Sheldon TA. A systematic review of compression treatment for venous leg ulcers. BMJ. 1997; 315 (7108):576–580

[47] Partsch H. Evidence based compression therapy. An initiative of the International Union of Phlebology. Vasa. 2004; 34:3–37

[48] O'Meara S, Cullum N, Nelson EA, Dumville JC. Compression for venous leg ulcers. Cochrane Database Syst Rev. 2012; 11: CD000265

[49] Partsch H. Compression therapy: clinical and experimental evidence. Ann Vasc Dis. 2012; 5(4):416–422

[50] Partsch H, Rabe E, Stemmer R. Compression therapy of the extremities. Paris: Editions Phlébologiques Francaises; 2000

[51] Nelson EA, Bell-Syer SE. Compression for preventing recurrence of venous ulcers. Cochrane Database Syst Rev. 2012(8): CD002303

[52] Nelson EA, Harper DR, Prescott RJ, Gibson B, Brown D, Ruckley CV. Prevention of recurrence of venous ulceration: randomized controlled trial of class 2 and class 3 elastic compression. J Vasc Surg. 2006; 44(4):803–808

[53] Badger CM, Peacock JL, Mortimer PS. A randomized, controlled, parallel-group clinical trial comparing multilayer bandaging followed by hosiery versus hosiery alone in the treatment of patients with lymphedema of the limb. Cancer. 2000; 88(12):2832–2837

[54] Mason M. Bandaging and subsequent elastic hosiery is more effective than elastic hosiery alone in reducing lymphoedema. Aust J Physiother. 2001; 47(2):153

[55] Jeanneret C, Aschwanden M, Staub D. Compression to prevent the postthrombotic syndrome. Phlebology. 2014; 29(1) suppl:71–77

[56] Bouman A, Cate-Hoek AT. Timing and duration of compression therapy after deep vein thrombosis. Phlebology. 2014; 29(1) suppl:78–82

[57] Amaragiri SV, Lees TA. Elastic compression stockings for prevention of deep vein thrombosis. Cochrane Database Syst Rev. 2000; 3(3):CD001484

[58] Kahn SR, Shapiro S, Wells PS, et al. SOX trial investigators. Compression stockings to prevent post-thrombotic syndrome: a randomised placebo-controlled trial. Lancet. 2014; 383 (9920):880–888

[59] Morris RJ, Woodcock JP. Evidence-based compression: prevention of stasis and deep vein thrombosis. Ann Surg. 2004; 239(2):162–171

[60] Kakkos SK, Caprini JA, Geroulakos G, Nicolaides AN, Stansby GP, Reddy DJ. Combined intermittent pneumatic leg compression and pharmacological prophylaxis for prevention of venous thromboembolism in high-risk patients. Cochrane Database Syst Rev. 2008; 4(4):CD005258

[61] Cesarone MR, Belcaro G, Agus G, et al. Management of superficial vein thrombosis and thrombophlebitis: status and expert opinion document. Angiology. 2007; 58 Suppl 1:7S–14S, discussion 14S–15S

[62] Rabe E, Partsch H, Jünger M, et al. Guidelines for clinical studies with compression devices in patients with venous disorders of the lower limb. Eur J Vasc Endovasc Surg. 2008; 35 (4):494–500

[63] Marston WA, Davies SW, Armstrong B, et al. Natural history of limbs with arterial insufficiency and chronic ulceration treated without revascularization. J Vasc Surg. 2006; 44 (1):108–114

[64] Silleran-Chassany J, Safran D. Prophylaxis of perioperative venous thrombosis: role of venous compression. Phlebology. 2000; 15:138–142

6 Endovenous Thermal Ablation

Amy R. Deipolyi, Gloria M. Martinez Salazar, and Felipe B. Collares

6.1 Introduction

Percutaneous endovascular thermal ablation (EVTA) for varicose veins has been proven to achieve results comparable to surgical venous stripping with less associated periprocedural morbidity and faster recovery, attractive features that allow patients to be treated in the outpatient setting. Its main advantages are that it allows for the exclusive use of local anesthetic, is minimally invasive, and is performed in the outpatient procedure setting with immediate patient discharge and ambulation. Choice of treatment for varicose veins depends on the presence or absence of venous reflux. There are several therapies available when reflux is not detected: sclerotherapy, transdermal laser treatment, ablation with echosclerotherapy, and ambulatory phlebectomy.[1,2,3]

When reflux is diagnosed, the classically performed intervention is saphenofemoral junction (SFJ) ligation with saphenous venous stripping. However, with the advent of ultrasound (US) and minimally invasive techniques resulting in a better understanding of anatomy and physiopathology of the venous disease, this approach has been increasingly replaced by EVTA under US guidance.[4,5]

Endovascular techniques for the treatment of varicose veins have emerged as a safe and effective alternative to traditional surgical therapy.[5] Recent clinical trials have shown equivalent long-term results compared to surgical vein stripping.[4,5] Practitioners involved in the care of these patients should have a thorough understanding of imaging aspects of venous insufficiency, as it relates to pre- and postprocedure patient evaluation, as well as to the performance of image-guided intervention.

6.2 Physics of Thermal Ablation

There are two different options of energy for thermal ablation of incompetent veins: radiofrequency ablation (RFA) or endovenous laser therapy (EVLT). RFA employs heat generated from high-frequency alternating current (AC), in the range of 350 to 500 kHz. In contrast to low-frequency AC or pulses of direct current (DC), RF current does not directly stimulate nerves and therefore can be used without general anesthesia. RFA requires a complete electrical circuit to conduct current, and therefore if monopolar electrodes are used, grounding pads are required. RF current can pass through tissue with ionic fluid. Tissue is not a perfect conductor, and therefore RF current induces resistive heating in tissue, termed the Joule effect. Within several millimeters of the RF electrode, direct heating occurs, whereas more peripheral areas may be heated due to thermal conduction. For vein RFA, bipolar electrodes are used to allow current flow between electrodes with focused and effective heating. Grounding pads are not needed.[6]

Laser, an acronym for light amplification by stimulated emission of radiation, involves the emission of single wavelength, monochromatic light with wavelengths ranging from short ultraviolet (< 420 nm) to long far-infrared (10,600 nm). Laser light consists of waves that are in phase; rays are parallel and nondiverging, producing stronger biologic effect than ordinary light of the same power.[7] Like all radiation, upon interacting with a target tissue, laser energy is absorbed, scattered, or reflected. Absorption allows for potentially therapeutic or damaging tissue effects. The extent of absorption depends on the amount of chromophores in a tissue, such as hemoglobin, melanin, proteins, and water, which absorb light of specific wavelengths.[7] After absorbing photons, chromophores are excited to higher energy states; upon de-excitation, energy is released back into the tissue, resulting in photochemical and photothermolytic changes. Photothermolysis is the primary mechanism of tissue effect in EVLT. The extent of laser absorption and consequent energy release depends on the chromophores present, which may be targeted with laser light of specific wavelengths.[7]

Scattering of laser light is also an important phenomenon determining its biologic effect. As it passes through matter, the light rays are scattered, reducing coherence and hence the effect of light on tissue. The extent of scattering determines the depth of laser light penetration, as tissue attenuates the incident beam. The amount of scattering is dependent on the nature of the chromophores and the wavelength of incident light. For example, light of longer wavelengths (1,470–1,500 nm) have much higher amounts of attenuation compared to light of shorter wavelengths (810–940 nm) in the vein wall, resulting in desirable greater tissue effect at the intended site of treatment.[7]

6.3 Biological Effects of Thermal Ablation

The cellular response of tissue to heating is well described. Prolonged heating at 42 to 45°C causes reversible sublethal cellular damage. At temperatures exceeding 50 to 60°C, irreversible damage, including cellular necrosis, occurs. At temperatures approaching 100°C, water vaporizes, producing steam and desiccating tissue. Tissue charring and possibly melting occurs above 300°C. Typically, outer vein wall temperatures during EVLT are of the order of 32 to 100°C, and intraluminal temperatures near the probes are on average 729°C.[7] In RFA, the vein wall is heated to 85°C with RF energy, which is delivered by temperature feedback–controlled catheter electrodes.[8]

Because blood, which normally fills the vein, and water, which is present in the vein wall and tissue surrounding the vein, cause a similar amount of attenuation of laser light, emptying the vein of blood is important for therapeutic effect, so that the biologic effect of the incident beam occurs on the vein wall itself rather than the blood within the vessel. This is accomplished during the procedure primarily by tumescent anesthesia, which constricts the vein by external compression and by inducing venospasm.[9]

Multiple theories exist to account for the tissue effects of EVLT (see the following list). The steam bubble theory focuses on the hyperechoic bubbles seen with US at the fiber tip during energy application, and suggests that these represent boiling blood that has an indirect effect, heating the vein wall. The heat pipe theory maintains that blood in immediate contact with the fiber becomes coagulated, forming a clot around the tip that acts as an insulating layer, trapping and then conducting heat to the vein wall. The direct contact theory suggests that maximal heat transfer to the vein wall occurs when the laser fiber contacts the vein wall. This happens frequently over the course of treatment, as the vein is typically relatively tortuous. Segments between these sites receive energy by conduction. Likely, the effect of EVLT on the vein wall is due to a combination of these proposed mechanisms.[7]

> ### Proposed Mechanisms of Action for EVLT[10]
>
> - Direct contact between the fiber tip and the vein wall.
> - Thermal interactions between the laser light and the vein wall:
>   - Direct absorption of the scattered light by the vein wall.
>   - Contact of heated blood with the vein wall.
> - Effect of steam bubbles produced by heated blood.
> - Effects of a carbonized blood layer attached to the fiber tip which absorbs light and becomes extremely hot damaging the vein wall.
> - Thermal injury of blood forming coagula within the vein lumen.

Histologic examination of veins removed immediately after thermal ablation demonstrates uneven vein wall destruction. The wall is perforated and ulcerated in areas of direct contact with the fiber tip, with relative sparing of the contralateral side. After 1 week, veins are thrombosed and demonstrate inflammatory tissue peripherally with migration of phagocytes and fibroblasts. There is uneven destruction of vein walls that is far more extensive than what is seen on veins harvested immediately after treatment. After 2 to 3 weeks, there is more organization of the perivenous inflammatory response, with scar tissue formation and proliferation of fibroblasts, myofibroblasts, and adventitial fibroblasts.[7]

In contrast to EVLT, RFA results in more homogeneous, circumferential destruction of the vein wall.[11] In RFA, temperature feedback–controlled catheter electrodes sustain thermal energy in the vein wall, inducing collagen contraction and endothelia denudation. This results in contraction of the vein wall, in contrast to EVLT which induces vein closure predominantly by occlusion.[8] RFA does not induce damage as extensive and transmural as EVLT, probably because the temperature feedback mechanism of the generator promotes a more circular, homogeneous distribution of thermal energy, compared with the laser fiber tip.[11] In addition, RF has characteristic low-temperature treatments (90–120°C), as compared to the laser, which can cause boiling, vaporizing, and carbonization of tissues (700–1,500°C).[12]

Table 6.1 Examples of commercially available laser devices

Laser λ	Device	Manufacturer
810 nm	Ceralas D15/810	Biolitec, East Longmeadow, MA
	Vari-Lase	Vascular Solutions, Minneapolis, MN
980 nm	Ceralas D, EVOLVE	Biolitec, East Longmeadow, MA
	Precision 980	Angiodynamics, Queensbury, NY
1,320 nm	CoolTouch CTEV	Cooltouch Corp., Roseville, CA
1,470 nm	VenaCure	Angiodynamics, Queensbury, NY
	ELVeS	Biolitec, East Longmeadow, MA

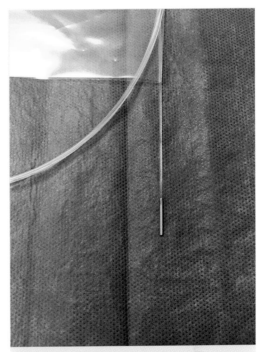

Fig. 6.1 Example of jacket-tip fiber (Angiodynamics NeverTouch Gold-Tip fiber).

6.4 Endovenous Laser Therapy

EVLT can be performed as an outpatient treatment using tumescent anesthesia and under US guidance. No preprocedural laboratory work-up is required. Lidocaine allergy is a relative contraindication to the procedure.

6.4.1 Equipment

Tumescent anesthesia can be delivered manually using a spinal needle, or with the use of a HK Klein Infiltration pump (HK Surgical Inc). The standard concentration of tumescent consists of normal saline and 1% lidocaine for a solution of 0.1% lidocaine mixed with normal saline. When performing bilateral EVTA, one must be cognizant of lidocaine toxicity and reduce the lidocaine concentration in the solution to 0.05%, which has been demonstrated to be safe in the outpatient setting.[13]

Several EVLT devices are available for clinical use, which are approved by Food and Drug Administration (▶ Table 6.1). Bare laser tip design has been traditionally used for different wavelengths, but because there is direct contact of the laser tip with the vein wall, associated vessel perforation occurs resulting in pain and bruising. In order to prevent that, other designs had been implemented since 2010, such as gold-tip, radial, and tulip-tip fibers. For example, covered or jacket-tip fibers eliminate the contact of the laser tip with the vessel wall, decreasing the risk of wall perforation and minimizing discomfort and bruising (▶ Fig. 6.1). US guidance is performed with grayscale and Doppler evaluation with linear transducers.

6.4.2 Treatment Protocols with Different Wavelengths

Endovenous laser obliteration employs one of several different wavelengths (810, 940, 980, 1,320, 1,470, and 1,500 nm) to produce thermal energy.[14] The thermal efficacy of EVLT is driven by the laser power, and different wavelengths deliver this energy to the vein wall differently: theoretically, the energy delivered by 1,470- to 1,500-nm wavelength light to the vein wall is much higher compared with 810- to 980-nm lasers, leading to greater selective destruction. This means that less power is needed by higher wavelengths in comparison with lower wavelengths to achieve the same thermal effect in the vein wall. Linear endovenous energy density (LEED) is the ratio of laser power to the velocity of the laser fiber pullback performed during the procedure and is measured in joules per centimeter (J/cm). Accordingly, lasers with higher wavelengths need a lower LEED (30–70 J/cm) to achieve the same results of lasers with lower wavelengths (70–120 J/cm).[7] When the laser power and the pullback velocity of the laser fiber are reported, the resulting LEED in J/cm serves as a parameter for reproducibility of the procedure, as other phlebologists can use the same protocol. In addition to wavelength, vein size also determines the amount of energy used because some authors may increase the LEED when treating veins with larger diameters.[10,15]

Longer wavelength devices of 1,470 to 1,500 nm have been proposed more recently because these wavelengths are preferentially absorbed by water, which would theoretically target the vein wall instead of blood. However, there is controversy regarding the power needed for treatment, and more research is needed to evaluate the efficacy and safety of these devices.[9] All current available laser devices have proven to be successful in closure of veins with high success rates (> 90%), independently of the wavelengths. There are few studies comparing different energy per centimeter of vein treated and protocols required for durable vein occlusion, with a suggested minimum threshold of 38 J/cm for veins < 6 mm in diameter and 63 J/cm in veins with a 10-mm diameter.[16]

6.4.3 Endovenous Laser Ablation Technique

Before the ablation, duplex US is performed to map incompetent sources of venous reflux, determining the incompetent portions of the great saphenous vein (GSV) starting at the SFJ, or the incompetent small saphenous vein (SSV) relative to the saphenopopliteal junction (SPJ).

Informed consent should be obtained, including a discussion of risks and benefits and other treatment alternatives. Although absolute contraindications for this procedure remain to be determined, relative contraindications for the EVTA as defined by the Society of Interventional Radiology guidelines include the following: pregnancy or nursing, obstructed deep venous system inadequate to support venous return after EVTA, liver dysfunction, allergy to lidocaine, severe uncorrectable coagulopathy, inability to wear compression stockings, inability to ambulate after the procedure, sciatic vein reflux, and nerve stimulator.[17]

The physician performing the procedure should wear gown and eye protection (including laser-specific attenuating glasses for the operator,

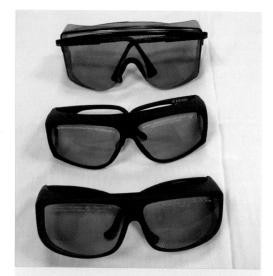

Fig. 6.2 Example of different protection glasses. The use of protective eyewear is required for every person in the procedure room while the laser is activated, including the operator, support staff, and patient.

patient, and staff; ▶ Fig. 6.2), and all staff in the procedural room should follow universal precautions. After consent is obtained, the patient is placed supine (for GSV treatment) or prone (for SSV treatment), and the region to be treated is sterilely prepared and isolated with sterile barriers (▶ Fig. 6.3). To maximize visualization of varicose veins, patients are placed in reverse Trendelenburg's position just before US-guided puncture.

US is used to select the appropriate venous access site, commonly around the knee for the GSV and midcalf for the SSV. Local anesthetic is delivered to the skin at the percutaneous access site (▶ Fig. 6.4), and the vein is punctured using a micropuncture venous access kit (▶ Fig. 6.5). Under real-time US guidance, the needle is advanced percutaneously into the vein lumen (▶ Fig. 6.6) and a 0.18-inch guidewire is advanced through the needle once intravascular position is confirmed (▶ Fig. 6.7). A small skin incision is performed at the puncture site and the needle is exchanged for the micropuncture sheath over the guidewire (▶ Fig. 6.8). The guidewire and the inner stiffener of the micropuncture sheath are then removed and a 0.35-inch guidewire is advanced through the sheath (▶ Fig. 6.9). The micropuncture sheath is then exchanged over the wire for the long vascular sheath through which the laser fiber will be inserted (▶ Fig. 6.10). The wire and inner stiffener of the vascular sheath are removed and the

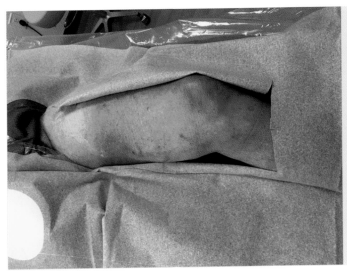

Fig. 6.3 Left lower extremity prepped and draped in a sterile fashion for great saphenous venous thermal ablation.

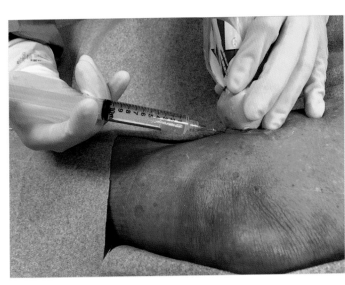

Fig. 6.4 Local anesthesia (1% lidocaine) is delivered to the skin over the great saphenous vein at the level of the left knee under ultrasound guidance.

position of the sheath is assessed by US (▶ Fig. 6.11). Under direct US guidance, the tip of the vascular sheath is positioned in the superficial venous system, typically 2 cm distal to the saphenofemoral or saphenopopliteal junction (▶ Fig. 6.12). At this point, the laser fiber is advanced through the vascular sheath and the position of the laser tip is confirmed by US (▶ Fig. 6.13). Confirmation of laser tip position in the superficial venous system distal to the saphenofemoral or saphenopopliteal junction before laser activation is crucial to avoid damage to the deep venous system.

At this point, the patient is then repositioned to a flat position to facilitate vein emptying, and tumescent anesthesia (0.1% lidocaine solution) is delivered under real-time US guidance in the perivenous sheath and surrounding subcutaneous tissue of the entire length of the anatomic region to be ablated (▶ Fig. 6.14). Successful ablation relies strongly on the use of tumescent anesthesia as well as the use of US to guide the position of the fiber within the vein. The rationale for the use of this type of anesthesia is based on the resistive heating of structures in direct contact with the electrode or laser, and the high temperatures attained to destroy the vein in situ. Besides its anesthetic effects, perivascular tumescent infiltration of lidocaine along the vein exerts two additional important functions: (1) it compresses and reduces the diameter of the vein, providing better vein wall apposition, and therefore circumferential

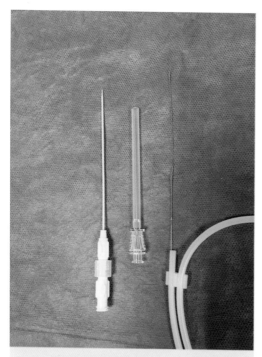

Fig. 6.5 Micropuncture venous access kit: micropuncture sheath, needle, and guidewire.

heating of the vein wall; and (2) it minimizes heat-related injury to adjacent tissues[4] (▶ Fig. 6.15).

During endovenous laser ablation, the thermal energy is delivered according to protocols inherent to the device utilized. Power delivered can be varied from 5 to 20 W. Energy per centimeter ranges from 20 to 100 J/cm, and energy may be delivered in a continuous or pulsed manner. Typically, the pullback of the laser fiber during venous ablation is performed at a 10 to 12 cm/minute rate and common protocols are continuous delivery of 80 J/cm at 12 W for 810-nm fibers and 70 J/cm at 14 W for 980-nm fibers.[18]

6.5 Endovenous Radiofrequency Ablation

6.5.1 Equipment

RFA includes the use of a generator with an especially devised disposable electrode catheter to deliver bipolar RF energy to the vein with temperatures not exceeding 120°C. The most commonly used device is the VNUS Ablation system (VNUS Medical Technologies), which uses a generator and bipolar catheter. This system is also called the

Closure procedure, and now newly named Venefit Targeted Endovenous Therapy (Covidien). This system uses the ClosureFast catheter, which heats the vein in 7-cm segments with 20-second treatment cycles resulting in venous occlusion. The temperature and power are continuously monitored during the procedure, heating the vein wall in a controlled fashion between 85 and 95°C. The ClosureFast catheter is also available with a 3-cm heating element, which is ideal for the treatment of shorter vein segments. The ClosureRFS Stylet is another available catheter option, which was specifically designed for the treatment of incompetent perforator and tributary veins (▶ Fig. 6.16).

6.5.2 Technique and Protocols

The same technique described for EVLT is utilized for RFA, with US-guided access of the GSV or SSV, followed by US-guided positioning of an RF catheter similar to positioning of the laser fiber. Tumescent anesthesia is delivered as described for EVLT. The vein is treated with segmental 3- or 7-cm ablations, depending on the selected catheter (▶ Fig. 6.16b). A 45-cm venous segment is usually ablated in 3 to 5 minutes with a 7-cm catheter.

6.6 Postprocedure Care and Follow-up

At the completion of the procedure, US evaluation of the SFJ or SPJ is performed to rule out deep vein thrombosis (DVT), followed by the placement of compression stocking (class 2) on the treated extremity. The patients are sent home after a brief recovery period.[14] Patients are instructed to wear compression stockings for 1 to 2 weeks. Ambulation is initiated immediately and should be encouraged during post-procedure use of compression stockings.[17]

Patients are routinely screened 1 to 2 weeks after endovenous treatment. Efficacy of endovenous ablation is assessed by US. Treated vessels are expected to contain echogenic thrombus, be non-compressible, and have no detectable blood flow. The presence of recanalization with blood flow in portions of a treated vessel may be due to patient noncompliance with stocking use following treatment. Endothermal heat-induced thrombosis (EHIT) is an expected finding in the treated GSV, and this type of thrombosis is typically hyperechoic, in contrast to de novo DVT, which is typically acutely hypoechoic. One useful classification

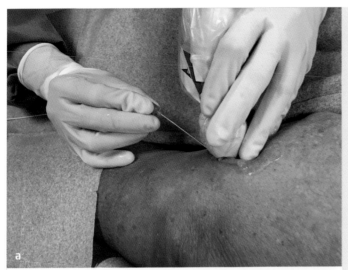

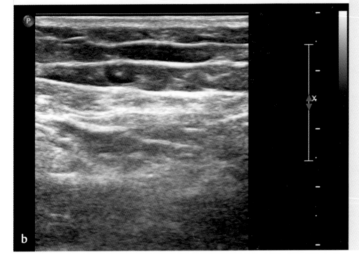

Fig. 6.6 Percutaneous access under ultrasound guidance. **(a)** The left great saphenous vein was punctured at the level of the knee. **(b)** Transverse ultrasound image demonstrating the intravascular position of the needle tip.

system described classes of EHIT in relation to the SFJ. Class 1 EHIT describes thrombosis to the level of the SJF. Class 2 describes nonocclusive thrombus extending into less than 50% the common femoral vein (CFV). Class 3 refers to nonocclusive thrombus extending more than 50% of the CFV lumen. Class 4 refers to thrombus occluding the CFV lumen. Class 1 EHIT may be managed conservatively, with monitoring by US. Class 2 and above are treated with anticoagulation, typically low-molecular-weight heparin, to prevent further propagation.[19, 20,21] When patients present complaining of significant lower extremity pain after endovascular therapy, US evaluation of the lower extremity is performed to exclude DVT, the most serious complication of EVTA.

6.7 Clinical Outcomes and Complications

Both techniques (RF and laser) are reported to provide successful closure of saphenous veins, with similar overall success and complications rates.[4] Prospective studies demonstrated that both methods effectively reduced symptoms of superficial venous insufficiency, but EVLT may be associated with greater bruising and discomfort in the perioperative period.[18] Reduced periprocedural pain and analgesic requirements are reported for patients undergoing closure with RF technique.[22,23] Durable vein occlusion was demonstrated in observational series with the use of laser to be more likely when energy delivery exceeded 80 J/cm.[24]

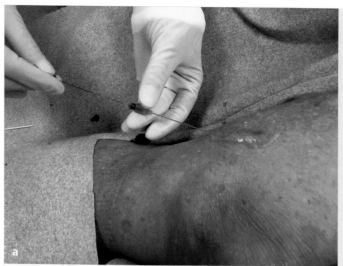

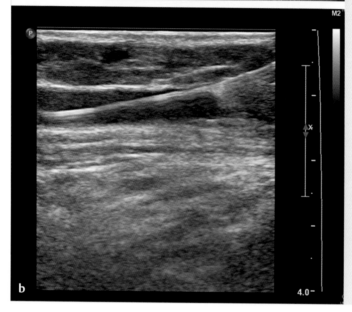

Fig. 6.7 (a) Introduction of the guidewire through the micropuncture needle into the great saphenous vein. (b) Longitudinal ultrasound image confirming intravascular position of the guidewire.

Success rates in the treatment of reflux of incompetent GSV have been described as more than 90% in early studies[25,26,27]; however, significant rates of paresthesia (5–19%) are reported in the literature. Pain, ecchymosis, induration, hematoma, and phlebitis are common adverse events, but they are usually self-limited. A recent randomized clinical trial demonstrated that endovenous laser ablation of the SSV had the same clinical benefits as conventional surgery, with less periprocedural morbidity and faster recovery.[28] In this study, resolution of SSV reflux was statistically significantly higher in the laser ablation group (96.2% of the patients) as compared to the surgical group (saphenopopliteal ligation followed by inversion stripping of the SSV). Minor complication rates were low in both groups, with higher incidence of paresthesias in the surgical group (26.4%) as compared with the laser ablation group (7.5%). Anatomical evaluation of the SSV and sural and tibial nerves demonstrates that the tibial nerve is at risk for post-EVTA paresthesias at the SPJ area, and the sural nerve is at risk for thermal damage in the distal two-thirds of the lower leg.[29]

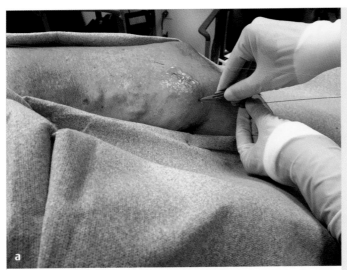

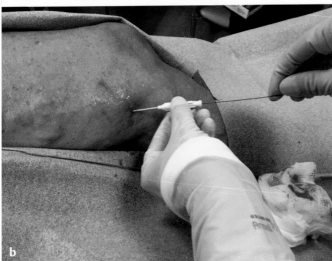

Fig. 6.8 (a) Small skin incision at the needle entry site at the skin. **(b)** Micropuncture sheath being advanced over the guidewire.

As mentioned, the most serious complication of venous thermal ablation is DVT. DVT is typically a result of propagation of thrombus from the treated GSV into the CFV at the SFJ, or from the treated SSV into the popliteal vein. Other complications include skin burns, discoloration, and hyperpigmentation in the course of the treated vein.[5] Damage to the sural nerve is particularly important when treating varicose veins at the level of the calf or SSV, where the sural nerve lies close and lateral to the SSV. In addition, due to the frequent anatomical variants at the SPJ level, a detailed evaluation of the SPJ with US is important for procedure planning and good outcome.

6.7.1 Additional Treatments

Ablation of Accessory Veins, Tributaries, and Perforators

After successful elimination of truncal reflux is performed with thermal ablation, there may still be a need to perform additional treatments for superficial varicosities, tributaries, and/or perforators. Treatment options include ambulatory phlebectomy, sclerotherapy, and thermal ablation. Timing of the additional treatments may vary, but a common approach is to perform these additional interventions at least 1 month after the EVTA

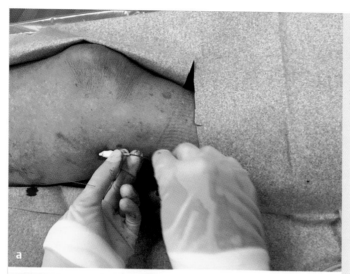

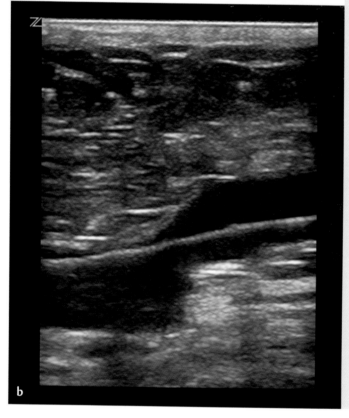

Fig. 6.9 (a) Introduction of the 0.35-inch guidewire through the micropuncture sheath into the great saphenous vein. (b) Longitudinal ultrasound image showing the guidewire crossing the saphenofemoral junction and entering the deep venous system.

procedure is completed and after evaluation with US to demonstrate successful closure of the main trunk and presence of additional incompetent tributaries. However, simultaneous EVTA treatment can be done in selected patients, particularly in the presence of an incompetent anterior or posterior accessory GSV (▶ Fig. 6.17). Furthermore, a recent study demonstrated the value of performing concomitant phlebectomy of large incompetent tributaries (>3 mm in diameter) in addition to RFA of the saphenous veins, with up to 83% of patients

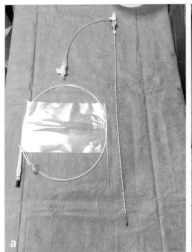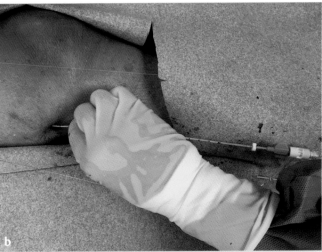

Fig. 6.10 The Angiodynamics endovenous laser ablation kit with the long vascular sheath and laser fiber. **(a)** Sheaths are available in different lengths and the centimeter marks help determining the total length of the treated vein segment and the pullback speed of the venous ablation. **(b)** The sheath is advanced into the great saphenous vein over the wire.

requiring additional phlebectomy due to persistent symptoms.[30]

Despite an ongoing debate regarding the value of perforator vein treatment in the setting of venous hypertension, surgical treatment with ligation of perforators has been considered the standard approach. More recent evidence on the use of 808-nm diode laser ablation for treatment of perforator veins demonstrated that this approach is a fast, safe, and effective option in vessels smaller than 6 mm in diameter. Only minor complications were observed in 11% of the patients, including phlebitis (8.8%), transitory paresthesia (1.5%), skin burns (4.8%), and pigmentation (3.7%).[31]

6.8 Additional Considerations

When endovenous thermal ablation fails to alleviate patient symptoms and clinical findings, or in cases of atypical presentation, alternative anatomic causes of lower extremity venous reflux should be pursued. Patients presenting with symptoms such as extensive edema, venous stasis dermatitis, and pain, which are out of proportion to initial US findings, or those with prior venous thrombosis or no explanation of their symptoms, may benefit from cross-sectional imaging of the venous outflow tracts to look for upstream venous obstruction.[32] The most common example of causes of central venous obstruction is May–Thurner anatomy with physiologically significant narrowing of the left common iliac vein by the overlying right common iliac artery (see Chapter 2, "Pathophysiology of Varicose Veins"). Other causes could include central obstructing masses or uterine fibroids, retroperitoneal fibrosis, and aberrant popliteal vein course causing compression by adjacent muscles (▶ Fig. 6.18). Such etiologies are best evaluating by computed tomography (CT) and magnetic resonance imaging (MRI), leading to other potential treatments, as endovenous ablation is not expected to provide effective treatment in these cases.

In conclusion, EVTA is a safe, minimally invasive procedure that has become the standard of care for varicose veins due to venous incompetence. Pre-procedural clinical and US evaluation is paramount to determine that the varicose veins are symptomatic and that they are associated with venous reflux. Doppler US is the essential first-line imaging tool, which demonstrates the presence of abnormal wave forms and increased valve closure time characteristic of incompetent veins. Additionally, US is key in the postprocedural evaluation for treatment success and to exclude the most worrisome complication, DVT.

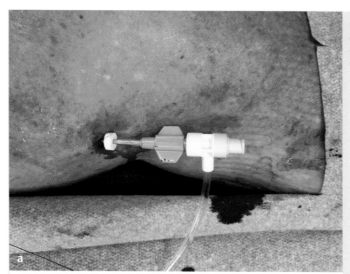

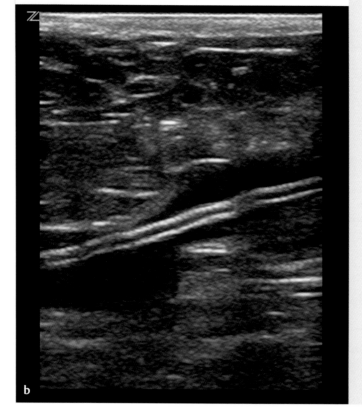

Fig. 6.11 (a) Vascular sheath in place. (b) Longitudinal ultrasound image showing the vascular sheath crossing the saphenofemoral junction.

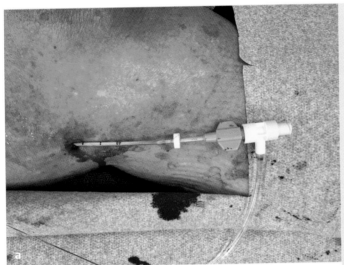

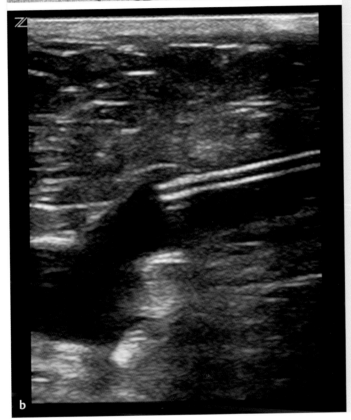

Fig. 6.12 (a) The vascular sheath is pulled back under ultrasound guidance and the tip is positioned 2 centimeters distal to the saphenofemoral junction. (b) Longitudinal ultrasound image confirming the position of the tip in the proximal great saphenous vein.

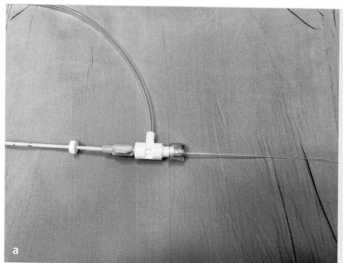

Fig. 6.13 **(a)** Laser fiber advanced into the vascular sheath. **(b)** Longitudinal ultrasound image demonstrating the tip of the laser fiber in the proximal great saphenous vein, distal to the saphenofemoral junction.

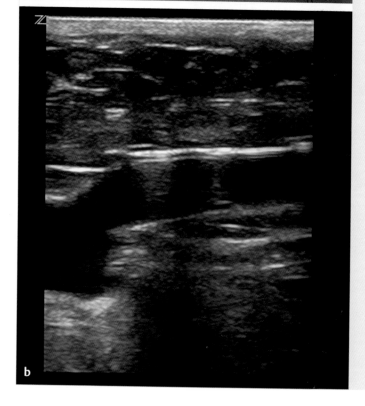

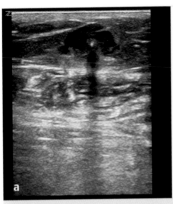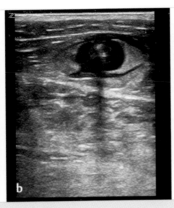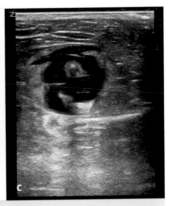

Fig. 6.14 **(a)** Transverse ultrasound images at the level of the distal thigh, **(b)** midthigh, and **(c)** proximal thigh after delivery of tumescent anesthesia.

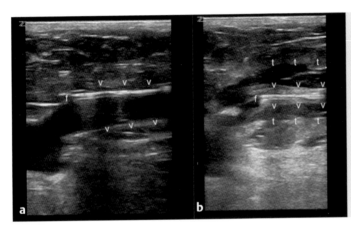

Fig. 6.15 Longitudinal ultrasound images of the proximal great saphenous vein **(a)** before and **(b)** after tumescent anesthesia. The tumescent anesthesia (t) compresses the vein wall (v) around the laser fiber (f), decreasing the diameter of the vessel.

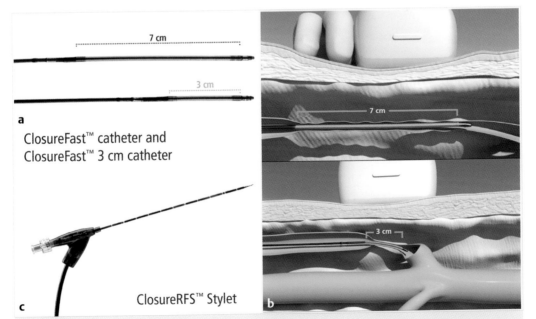

ClosureFast™ catheter and ClosureFast™ 3 cm catheter

ClosureRFS™ Stylet

Fig. 6.16 The Venefit Targeted Endovenous Therapy (Covidien) system with the ClosureFast catheters available in different sizes **(a)**. The vein can be treated in 3- or 7-cm segments **(b)**. The ClosureRFS Stylet **(c)** designed for the treatment of incompetent perforator and tributary veins. (Courtesy of Medtronic. © Covidien. All rights reserved)

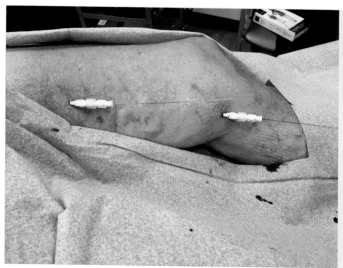

Fig. 6.17 Incompetent great saphenous vein (GSV) and anterior accessory great saphenous vein. The GSV was accessed at the level of the knee and the anterior accessory GSV was accessed at the level of the mid/upper thigh and treated with EVTA.

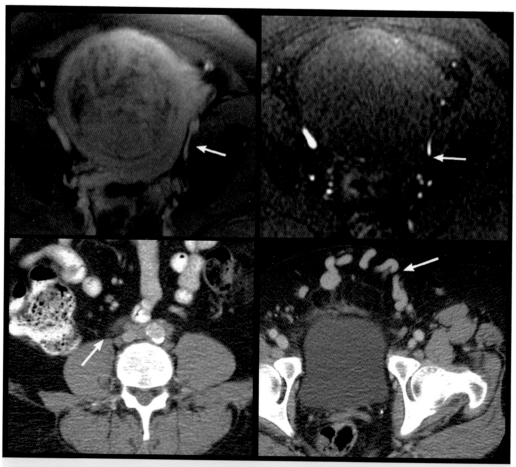

Fig. 6.18 Examples of central venous obstruction leading to chronic lower extremity venous disease. The top row shows MRI demonstrating compression of the left external iliac vein by a fibroid uterus in a 40-year-old woman with chronic left leg pain and weakness. The bottom row shows CT images of chronic left common iliac stenosis and left lower extremity DVT from retroperitoneal fibrosis in a 68-year-old woman presenting with chronic left lower extremity fatigue, pain, varicose veins, and DVT. The bottom left image shows tight stenosis of the inferior vena cava (IVC), with resultant venous collaterals (arrow) seen in the bottom right image.

References

[1] Bergan JJ, Sparks SR, Owens EL, Kumins NH. Growing the vascular surgical practice: venous disorders. Cardiovasc Surg. 2001; 9(5):431–435

[2] Campbell B. New treatments for varicose veins. BMJ. 2002; 324(7339):689–690

[3] Weiss RA, Dover JS. Leg vein management: sclerotherapy, ambulatory phlebectomy, and laser surgery. Semin Cutan Med Surg. 2002; 21(1):76–103

[4] Min RJ, Khilnani N, Zimmet SE. Endovenous laser treatment of saphenous vein reflux: long-term results. J Vasc Interv Radiol. 2003; 14(8):991–996

[5] Mundy L, Merlin TL, Fitridge RA, Hiller JE. Systematic review of endovenous laser treatment for varicose veins. Br J Surg. 2005; 92(10):1189–1194

[6] Brace CL. Radiofrequency and microwave ablation of the liver, lung, kidney, and bone: what are the differences? Curr Probl Diagn Radiol. 2009; 38(3):135–143

[7] Vuylsteke ME, Mordon SR. Endovenous laser ablation: a review of mechanisms of action. Ann Vasc Surg. 2012; 26 (3):424–433

[8] Weiss RA. Comparison of endovenous radiofrequency versus 810 nm diode laser occlusion of large veins in an animal model. Dermatol Surg. 2002; 28(1):56–61

[9] Mordon SR, Vuylsteke ME. Varicose veins: endovenous laser treatment. In: Raulin C, Karsai S, eds. Laser and IPL Technology in Dermatology and Aesthetic Medicine. Berlin: Springer; 2010:211–225

[10] Neumann HA, van Gemert MJ. Ins and outs of endovenous laser ablation: afterthoughts. Lasers Med Sci. 2014; 29 (2):513–518

[11] Schmedt CG, Sroka R, Steckmeier S, et al. Investigation on radiofrequency and laser (980 nm) effects after endoluminal treatment of saphenous vein insufficiency in an ex-vivo model. Eur J Vasc Endovasc Surg. 2006; 32(3):318–325

[12] García-Madrid C, Pastor Manrique JO, Gómez-Blasco F, Sala Planell E. Update on endovenous radio-frequency closure ablation of varicose veins. Ann Vasc Surg. 2012; 26(2):281–291

[13] Janne d'Othée B, Faintuch S, Schirmang T, Lang EV. Endovenous laser ablation of the saphenous veins: bilateral versus unilateral single-session procedures. J Vasc Interv Radiol. 2008; 19(2, Pt 1):211–215

[14] Ombrellino M, Kabnick LS. Varicose vein surgery. Semin Intervent Radiol. 2005; 22(3):185–194

[15] Almeida JI, Raines JK. Radiofrequency ablation and laser ablation in the treatment of varicose veins. Ann Vasc Surg. 2006; 20(4):547–552

[16] van den Bos RR, Proebstle TM. The state of the art of endothermal ablation. Lasers Med Sci. 2014; 29(2):387–392

[17] Khilnani NM, Grassi CJ, Kundu S, et al. Cardiovascular Interventional Radiological Society of Europe, American College of Phlebology, and Society of Interventional Radiology Standards of Practice Committees. Multi-society consensus quality improvement guidelines for the treatment of lower-extremity superficial venous insufficiency with endovenous thermal ablation from the Society of Interventional Radiology,

Cardiovascular Interventional Radiological Society of Europe, American College of Phlebology and Canadian Interventional Radiology Association. J Vasc Interv Radiol. 2010; 21(1):14–31

[18] Nordon IM, Hinchliffe RJ, Brar R, et al. A prospective double-blind randomized controlled trial of radiofrequency versus laser treatment of the great saphenous vein in patients with varicose veins. Ann Surg. 2011; 254(6):876–881

[19] Kabnick LS. Complications of endovenous therapies: statistics and treatment. Vascular. 2006; 14:S31–S32

[20] Dexter D, Kabnick L, Berland T, et al. Complications of endovenous lasers. Phlebology. 2012; 27 Suppl 1:40–45

[21] Anwar MA, Lane TR, Davies AH, Franklin IJ. Complications of radiofrequency ablation of varicose veins. Phlebology. 2012; 27 Suppl 1:34–39

[22] Goode SD, Chowdhury A, Crockett M, et al. Laser and radiofrequency ablation study (LARA study): a randomised study comparing radiofrequency ablation and endovenous laser ablation (810 nm). Eur J Vasc Endovasc Surg. 2010; 40(2):246–253

[23] Gale SS, Lee JN, Walsh ME, Wojnarowski DL, Comerota AJ. A randomized, controlled trial of endovenous thermal ablation using the 810-nm wavelength laser and the ClosurePLUS radiofrequency ablation methods for superficial venous insufficiency of the great saphenous vein. J Vasc Surg. 2010; 52(3):645–650

[24] Sadick NS, Wasser S. Combined endovascular laser with ambulatory phlebectomy for the treatment of superficial venous incompetence: a 2-year perspective. J Cosmet Laser Ther. 2004; 6(1):44–49

[25] Min RJ, Khilnani NM, Golia P. Duplex ultrasound evaluation of lower extremity venous insufficiency. J Vasc Interv Radiol. 2003; 14(10):1233–1241

[26] Meissner MH. Lower extremity venous anatomy. Semin Intervent Radiol. 2005; 22(3):147–156

[27] Browse NL, Burnand KG, Thomas ML. Diseases of the Veins: Pathology, Diagnosis, and Treatment. London: Edward Arnold; 1988

[28] Samuel N, Carradice D, Wallace T, Mekako A, Hatfield J, Chetter I. Randomized clinical trial of endovenous laser ablation versus conventional surgery for small saphenous varicose veins. Ann Surg. 2013; 257(3):419–426

[29] Kerver AL, van der Ham AC, Theeuwes HP, et al. The surgical anatomy of the small saphenous vein and adjacent nerves in relation to endovenous thermal ablation. J Vasc Surg. 2012; 56(1):181–188

[30] Harlander-Locke M, Jimenez JC, Lawrence PF, Derubertis BG, Rigberg DA, Gelabert HA. Endovenous ablation with concomitant phlebectomy is a safe and effective method of treatment for symptomatic patients with axial reflux and large incompetent tributaries. J Vasc Surg. 2013; 58(1):166–172

[31] Corcos L, Pontello D, DE Anna D, et al. Endovenous 808-nm diode laser occlusion of perforating veins and varicose collaterals: a prospective study of 482 limbs. Dermatol Surg. 2011; 37(10):1486–1498

[32] Meissner MH, Eklof B, Smith PC, et al. Secondary chronic venous disorders. J Vasc Surg. 2007; 46 Suppl S:68S–83S

7 Sclerotherapy

Ian M. Brennan

7.1 Introduction

Venous sclerotherapy is the targeted injection of a chemical irritant into the lumen of a vein to produce inflammation, occlusion, and eventual fibrosis. A small amount of damage to the vein wall can induce intravascular thrombosis; however, in the presence of an intact endothelial lining, the vessel will usually recanalize over time.[1] In contrast, the goal of sclerotherapy is to cause irreversible complete endothelial cellular damage, full vessel wall destruction with permanent obliteration of the vascular lumen (endosclerosis), eventually resulting in a residual fibrous cord (endofibrosis). Sclerotherapy is indicated in the treatment of a wide range of abnormal veins—from small telangiectasias to incompetent truncal saphenous veins. The availability of multiple agents and variable drug concentrations and ability to modify agent composition (liquid or foam) combine to make sclerotherapy a powerful treatment modality in the management of varicose vein disease.

7.2 Indications

Injection sclerotherapy is indicated in a wide range of venous disease processes, including treatment of incompetent truncal and other large varicose veins, incompetent perforating veins, reticular and telangiectatic veins, and venous malformations. Although beyond the scope of this chapter, its use extends to treat other medical conditions, including submucosal esophageal and gastric varices, scrotal varicoceles, vulvar varicosities, hemorrhoids, hygromas, lymphatic cysts, and Baker's cysts.[2]

Liquid sclerotherapy is considered the treatment of choice for small reticular veins and telangiectasias—CEAP (clinical, etiology, anatomy, pathophysiology) class C1 (see Chapter 3, "The Clinical Exam," for the CEAP classification system).[2] Foam sclerotherapy is also the treatment of choice in suitable CEAP class C2 varicose veins.[2] In addition, along with more established surgical and endovascular ablative techniques, studies have proven foam sclerotherapy to be a safe, effective, and affordable treatment for saphenous vein incompetence.[3,4,5]

7.3 Contraindications

Absolute contraindications to injection sclerotherapy include known allergy to the proposed sclerosant agent, acute deep venous thrombosis, active infectious process involving the area to be treated, and prolonged immobility which increases the risk of postprocedure deep vein thrombosis (DVT). In addition, when the use of foam sclerotherapy is planned, the presence of a symptomatic right-to-left cardiac shunt should be considered an absolute contraindication due to the increased risk of paradoxical air embolism, a complication discussed later in this chapter.[2]

Postsclerotherapy compression is important in reducing thrombophlebitis, and therefore, a patient's inability to wear compression stockings (as exists with significant lower extremity arterial insufficiency) should be considered a relative contraindication.[6] Other relative contraindications should be considered on a case-by-case basis and include pregnancy, inability to ambulate, prothrombotic syndromes, and multiple drug allergies. More specifically, care must be taken in patients taking the estrogen receptor antagonist tamoxifen as the incidence of superficial thrombophlebitis is higher.[7] Also, patients taking the acetaldehyde dehydrogenase inhibitor disulfiram should avoid polidocanol [POL] because it contains ethyl alcohol (see later).[6] Finally, a thorough risk/benefit discussion should also be had with any patient who had neurologic symptoms following prior administration of foam sclerotherapy.[8]

7.4 Sclerosing Agents and Mechanisms of Action

Sclerosants are designed to irreversibly damage the vascular endothelium but are also capable of damaging surrounding tissue. This endothelial destruction is dependent on the administered sclerosant dose and the contact time between the agent and the endothelial layer. The ideal sclerosing agent would cause rapid full-thickness vascular wall damage with minimal thrombus formation, be minimally toxic to adjacent structures, be hypoallergenic, and not result in hyper- or hypopigmentation of the overlying skin.

Unfortunately, such an agent does not exist; however, the careful use of modern sclerosant medications in the appropriate concentration and form will usually result in a safe and effective treatment. Effective sclerotherapy is dependent on damage of the entire vessel wall, not just the endothelial layer. Rapid endothelial regeneration and migration can occur if the surrounding vascular smooth muscle cells are left intact, leading to eventual vessel recanalization.[9] In vitro work with the two most widely used detergent sclerosant agents (0.3% POL and 0.1% sodium tetradecyl sulfate [STS]) has demonstrated cell death in cultured endothelial cells within 15 minutes of incubation.[10] In vivo, endothelial cell death causes exposure of collagen fibers, which in turn activates the intrinsic blood coagulation pathway. As a result, thrombus generation always occurs to some degree following sclerotherapy but can be problematic, leading to excessive inflammation and eventual recanalization. Thrombus generated following full-thickness endothelial damage has different properties to conventional intravascular thrombus, including a higher white blood cell count and inflammatory infiltration of the vessel wall, making it strongly adherent.[11] It is important to stress that sclerosant agents do not mediate their effects through the generation of thrombosis but rather via direct vessel wall injury.

Studies have shown that patients receiving systemic anticoagulation medications had no reduction in treatment efficacy following foam sclerotherapy.[12] Similarly, the addition of heparin to the detergent sclerosant STS did not reduce its treatment efficacy.[13] Sclerosing agents can be broadly classified into three categories based on the mechanism of cell damage: detergent-based sclerosants, hyperosmotic agents, and chemical irritants. Agents are usually administered individually but may be combined for a particular clinical indication.[14]

7.4.1 Detergent Solutions

In worldwide use since the 1930s, detergent-based agents are now the most popular sclerosant class in the treatment of varicose vein disease. Above a certain concentration, detergent molecules organize themselves into micelles, which, via a number of mechanisms including a process called protein theft denaturation, cause disruption of the cell surface membrane through interference of cell surface lipids.[15] Irreversible cell changes occur within minutes of contact. Agents include sodium morrhuate, ethanolamine oleate, and the two most widely used agents—STS and POL. Sodium morrhuate (Scleromate, Palisades Pharmaceuticals) and ethanolamine oleate (Ethamolin, QOL Medical) are agents which were in use prior to the establishment of the Food and Drug Administration (FDA) in the United States and were accordingly "grandfathered in" primarily for use in the treatment of esophageal varices. Their use in the treatment of lower extremity varicose veins is not routinely recommended given reported skin necrosis with extravasation of both agents and the relatively high incidence of severe anaphylactic reactions with sodium morrhuate.[1] Given the modern widespread use of STS and POL, we will focus on these agents in more detail.

Sodium Tetradecyl sulfate

STS (sodium-1 isobutyl-4-ethyloctyl sulfate; Sotradecol, Bioniche Pharma Group, Inverin, Co.; Thromboject, Omega Laboratories; Trombovar, Laboratoires Innothéra; Fibro-Vein, STD Pharmaceutical Products) is a long-chain fatty acid salt and has been in commercial use in the United States since before the establishment of the FDA in 1938. Accordingly, this agent was also "grandfathered in" and as a result it was never objectively evaluated for its role in venous reflux disease. Nevertheless, STS has been in widespread use for more than 60 years and has a proven track record in terms of both safety and efficacy.[15] It is commercially available in concentrations ranging from 0.2 to 3% and comes as a clear nonviscous fluid. STS is a powerful sclerosant agent and has been shown to produce maceration of the endothelium within 1 second of exposure.[16] STS is approximately two to three times as potent as POL at the same concentration. The maximal advised sessional dose varies between manufacturers, with a volume of 4 mL of 3% STS recommended by STD Pharmaceutical Products but up to 10 mL of 3% solution is recommended by Bioniche Pharma Group.[17,18] Larger volumes may be appropriate at lower concentrations. For adverse reactions, see later.

Polidocanol

POL (laurel macro gel 400 laureth-9; Aethoxysklerol, Asclera Kreussler & Co., GMBH) is a synthetic long-chain fatty acid nonionic detergent with local anesthetic properties. It was originally marketed in 1936 as a topical anesthetic agent, but its use as a vascular sclerosant did not start until the 1960s.[1] It is marketed as an injectable sclerosant and is available in a number of different concentrations ranging from 0.25 to 4%. A dose limit of 2 mg per kg body weight is described (10 mL of 1% solution in a 50-kg patient).[15] However, other authors have reported higher volumes and concentrations with no ill effects.[19] It was approved by the FDA in 2010 for use in the United States in treatment of telangiectasias and reticular veins only. Although considered a weaker sclerosant agent than STS, POL is equally efficacious as a venous sclerosant with a generally better safety profile. It is painless to inject, and allergic reactions have rarely been reported. For adverse reactions, see later.

Detergent Foams

Agitation of liquid detergent sclerosant with a gas results in creation of foam. When injected into the vein lumen, this detergent foam has the ability to displace blood rather than mix with it and thus maximizes endothelial surface contact area and time, all with a lower required volume of liquid solution. It should be noted, however, that if the injected foam volume is too small for the vein diameter, the foam may simply float on the intravascular blood contacting only the nondependent endothelial surface. Cabrera et al first described the use "sclerofoam" in the 1990s, building on much earlier work from Foote in 1944 and Orbach and Petretti in 1950.[20,21,22] A simple technique to produce a durable foam was described by Tessari et al using a three-way connecter.[23] They found a ratio of one part liquid sclerosant to four parts air to be optimal in generating a dense, durable foam. Carbon dioxide, oxygen, and room air have all been used in foam generation, with no clear consensus on the optimal sclerosant to air/gas ratio.[24] As carbon dioxide is denser than room air, foam bubbles are smaller in size. This is advantageous as smaller bubble size translates to increase in surface area of the sclerosant and less blood mixing. CO_2-based foam, however, degrades more quickly than room air and must be injected rapidly following generation. Some authors have shown that when high-volume foam administration is performed, the use of CO_2-based foam appears to reduce early-onset reversible neurologic side effects when compared with room air.[25] Others have shown no difference in neurologic effects between air-based foam and that generated with a 30% O_2/70% CO_2 gas mixture

when used at lower foam volumes.[26] Although there is no evidence-based limit for the maximum volume of foam administered per session, the European Consensus on Foam Sclerotherapy considered 10 mL as safe as an expert opinion.[8]

7.4.2 Hyperosmotic Agents

Sclerosing agents in this class include hypertonic saline (HS), sodium salicylate (Saliject, Omega Laboratories), and formulations of dextrose and HS (Sclerodex, Omega Laboratories). Concentrated hyperosmolar solutions are thought to partially denature cell surface proteins through dehydration but require several minutes to exert their full effect, especially as full-thickness vein wall destruction is required. Studies have shown that endothelial cell death using HS occurs only after 3 minutes of contact time and treated endothelial cells do not detach into the vessel lumen as seen following administration of detergent-based sclerosant agents.[16] Accordingly, these agents are primarily suited for small vessels such as extremity telangiectasias and small reticular veins.

HS is a weak sclerosant in use since the 1920s. Currently, HS is only FDA approved for use in the United States as an abortifacient and accordingly its use is considered off label for venous sclerosis. The principal advantage of HS over detergent-based sclerosant agents is the absence of allergic reactions when given in its pure form. The major drawback of HS is pain on injection and the potential for extensive tissue necrosis with even a small amount of extravascular administration.[6] Administration has also been associated with severe muscle cramping. In addition, hyperosmotic agents cause erythrocyte hemolysis, which can lead to punctate hyperpigmentation. Other potential complications include hematuria, renal cortical necrosis, and hypertension.[6]

Practitioners have described diluting the HS solution with lidocaine to vary the HS solution between 18 and 30% depending on vein caliber.[27] The role of HS in venous disease is now generally limited to injection of telangiectasias in patients with a documented allergy to detergent sclerosant agents. HS with dextrose formulations are believed to be less painful to inject and are associated with less muscle cramping.[28] Sodium salicylate is usually diluted with lidocaine to reduce pain but is again associated with muscle cramping and risk of necrosis if extravasation occurs.[6]

7.4.3 Chemical Irritants

Agents in this category include denatured alcohol, polyiodinated iodine (Sclerodine, Omega Laboratories; Variglobin, Globopharm), and chromated glycerin (Sclérémo, Laboratories Bailleul; Chromex, Omega Laboratories) and act directly on endothelial cells, likely via disruption of intercellular binding proteins. Glycerin is a mild sclerosant that rarely causes hyperpigmentation or necrosis and is hypoallergenic in its pure form.[29] Although a direct chemical irritant, it likely also exerts an osmotic effect. Given its high viscosity, it can be difficult to inject through a narrow gauge needle and is often diluted with lidocaine. The addition of chromium increases the sclerosant potency and prevents hematuria, which can be seen with use of glycerin alone in high doses.[30] It has a very good side-effect profile; however, its use is cautioned in diabetic patients because there is a potential risk of hyperglycemia.[6]

7.5 Sclerotherapy Technique

As with any medical intervention, a thorough informed consent is required outlining the risks and benefits of the proposed procedure. It is important to stress the realistic goals of treatment and to explain from the outset that short- and medium-term follow-up sessions may be required. Specific complications related to injection sclerotherapy should be discussed (see later). Increasing the concentration and volume of administered sclerosant will increase the likelihood of treatment success; however, the risk of complications also rises. Ideally, the minimum concentration and volume of agent should be delivered to cause irreversible vascular damage while sparing the surrounding tissues.

7.5.1 Liquid Sclerotherapy for Reticular Veins and Telangiectasias

Technique

Most practitioners advise against shaving the treatment area on the day of the procedure because this may lead to stinging on application of alcohol-based antiseptic solutions. Application of moisturizing cream is also discouraged as it renders the skin slippery and difficult to make taut during vein cannulation.[6] Photographs should be taken of the lower extremities to act as a baseline prior to initiation of a treatment regimen. The treated body part should be placed in a horizontal position as gravity-aided dilatation is not needed in treatment of reticular or telangiectatic veins (and may worsen intravascular thrombosis). It is very helpful to use an adjustable tilt table which allows positioning of the patient at a comfortable height for the operator but also to have the ability to place the patient in Trendelenburg's or reverse Trendelenburg's position as required. The area is cleansed using an alcohol wipe, which in addition to an antiseptic effect also renders the skin somewhat more transparent and may even cause a degree of vasodilatation.[6] Many operators find the use of magnification with or without polarized light greatly beneficial in visualization of small telangiectasias and reticular veins (▶ Fig. 7.1).

The use of small caliber (30 G) needles is advised to minimize trauma to the vein wall. Some authors advocate the use of even smaller (32–33 G) needles for very small vessels, but such needles tend to bend easily.[31] The needle is connected to either a 3 or 1 mL syringe, sometimes via a short segment of kink resistant connecting tubing. It should be remembered that much higher pressures are generated with use of small-volume syringes and care must be taken to avoid vessel injury and extravasation. As a general rule, the telangiectatic vessel should be injected slowly and with the least force required to fill the vessel lumen. Gentle tension should be applied to the skin to stabilize the target vessel. As telangiectasias lie within the dermis, it is important to be as superficial as possible. Most practitioners find it helpful to bend the needle slightly and to enter the vessel with the bevel facing upward, almost parallel to the skin surface (▶ Fig. 7.2). Some physicians advocate injection of a minute amount of air to confirm intravascular position prior to injection of sclerosant, the so-

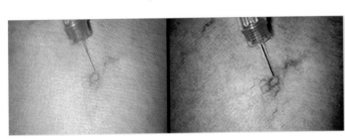

Fig. 7.1 Telangiectatic vein appearance using polarized light. (Reprinted with permission from Syris Scientific.)

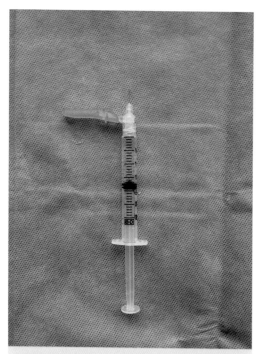

Fig. 7.2 Liquid sclerotherapy: 3-mL syringe and a 30-G needle with 140-degree angulation to aid cannulation of superficial telangiectatic veins.

called air block technique.[32] Alternatively, aspiration of a small amount of blood and rapid linear blanching of the target vein on injection of sclerosant also indicates satisfactory intravascular position. Generalized, nonlinear whitening of the tissue or burning pain is indicative of extravascular position of the needle, and injection should be stopped immediately.

The volume administered per injection should be small to reduce unwanted side effects. As a general rule, injection should be stopped when blood displacement is no longer seen. Detergent sclerosant injection volumes of less than 0.2 mL in telangiectatic veins and 0.5 mL in reticular veins are recommended[2] (▶ Table 7.1).

Following injection, the vessel may go into spasm and there is often mild perivascular edema.

Erythema and urticaria may also be seen in the treated area, and if the patient complains of pruritus, the application of topical steroid cream may be of benefit prior to placing the compressive dressing.[6]

7.5.2 Foam Sclerotherapy for Varicose Veins and Truncal Varicosities

Foam Generation

Several methods exist to generate injectable detergent foam, including simply shaking a syringe to the use of an automated foaming device (Turbofoam, Kreussler Pharma). As mentioned earlier, the Tessari method is a simple and reproducible way of generating a viscous, finely bubbled, and homogeneous foam.[23] It involves connecting a 10-mL syringe containing the desired liquid sclerosant (and diluent if required) to another 10-mL syringe containing a known volume of CO_2 gas or room air via a three-way stopcock. Some authors have described the use of a 5-μm filter placed between the syringes to improve foam quality.[33] The two syringes are then injected back and forth via the stopcock 10 to 15 times, generating a homogeneous foam (▶ Fig. 7.3). As originally described and mentioned earlier, the ratio of liquid sclerosant to air or gas is 1:4.[23] No adverse effects have been attributed to the use of nonsterile room air.[34] It is advisable to inject the foam quickly after it is created for optimal results because foam degrades after about 2 minutes.

Technique

As with liquid sclerotherapy, most practitioners now perform foam sclerotherapy with the patient in the recumbent position. A tilt table is of benefit to temporarily position the patient in a reverse Trendelenburg's position to aid venous distention when cannulating smaller varicosities. Following injection, elevation of the legs above the level of

Table 7.1 Suggested polidocanol (POL) and sodium tetradecyl sulfate (STS) concentrations and volume per injection point for liquid sclerotherapy depending on target vessel size[1,2]

Target vessel	% concentration of POL	% concentration of STS	Volume/injection point
Telangiectasias	0.25 to 0.5%	0.1 to 0.2%	Up to 0.2 mL
Reticular veins	0.5 to 1%	0.2 to 0.5%	Up to 0.5 mL
Varicose veins	1 to 3 %	1 to 3 %	Up to 2.0 mL

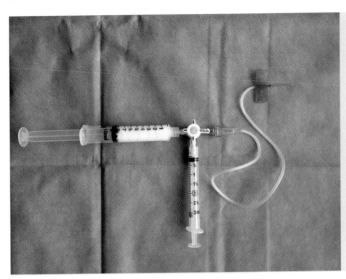

Fig. 7.3 Foam sclerotherapy. Foam generation using the Tessari technique.

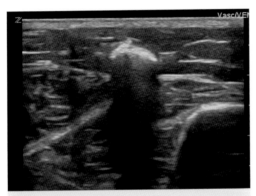

Fig. 7.4 Appearance of injected 0.5% STS foam in the distal GSV. Note hyperechoic vessel lumen with shadowing deep to the vessel.

the heart is important because it minimizes venous distension and maximizes surface contact.

When injecting foam, ultrasound is an excellent modality to guide vessel cannulation and monitor foam distribution due the inherent sound wave scatter generated by the multiple air/liquid interfaces. Intravascular foam has a characteristic echogenic appearance on ultrasound (▶ Fig. 7.4). The needle diameter for administration of foam sclerotherapy should not be narrower than 25 G to prevent degradation of the foam quality and maintain the microbubble suspension.

It is important to establish all required intravascular needle access prior to foam administration because, once injected, foam will spread into more superficial branches, making further ultrasound-guided venous access difficult to perform. Many authors advocate use a short 18-G cannula for foam injection of truncal varicosities to ensure stable intravenous position.[33] When used to treat the great saphenous vein, this cannula is usually placed in the lower third of the thigh. Smaller caliber (23 G) butterfly needles are then used to cannulate more superficial varicosities. Although practice varies, the smaller varicosities are usually injected first with foam, prior to treatment of the main great saphenous vein. When performing ultrasound-guided foam sclerotherapy of the great saphenous vein, many authors advocate that the first injection should be located 10 to 20 cm below the saphenofemoral junction with positioning of the patient in the Trendelenburg's position. This optimizes filling of the saphenous trunk up to the saphenofemoral junction but avoids excessive passage of foam into the deep veins through distal perforators.[8] Immediate contraction of the target vessel following administration of foam is usually observed and may be used as a treatment end point.

Most practitioners advocate periodic active ankle dorsiflexion between injections to rapidly flush foam from the deep system. Usually, 6 to 8 mL of 3% detergent foam is required for the thigh segment of the GSV. There are little data on the acceptable upper limit for foam volume in a given treatment session but higher volumes may produce higher rates of DVT.[35] Expert opinion established 10 mL of foam as a safe upper limit, as transient side effects and thromboembolic complications increase above this amount.[8,36] It is not recommended to administer more than 2 mL of foam per injection, and to deliver it slowly over 10 to 15 seconds.[2]

Table 7.2 Suggested polidocanol (POL) and sodium tetradecyl sulfate (STS) concentrations for foam sclerotherapy depending on target vessel size[1,2]

Target vessel	% concentration of POL	% concentration of STS
Reticular veins	Up to 0.5%	Up to 0.5%
Tributary varicose veins	Up to 2%	Up to 1%
Saphenous veins < 4 mm	Up to 1%	Up to 1%
Saphenous veins > 4 and < 8 mm	1 to 3%	1 to 3%
Saphenous veins > 8 mm	3%	3%

Guidelines on the suggested concentration of the two most commonly used detergent sclerosant agents were created by 23 European phlebologic societies in 2012 and are summarized in ▶ Table 7.1 and ▶ Table 7.2.[2]

7.6 Postprocedure Care and Follow-up

Patient follow-up after sclerotherapy is critical to assess treatment response, gauge patient satisfaction, detect and treat early complications, and perform outcome data collection for clinical research and audit. As mentioned, before and after photographs can be useful in documenting treatment response and also allow blinded third party review at a later date for research and quality assurance purposes.[37]

Postprocedure care following foam sclerotherapy of truncal varicose veins is broadly similar to that performed following endovenous ablation. Sterile adhesive dressings should be placed over skin puncture points followed by an elasticized cohesive bandage. A roll of gauze may be placed directly over the vein and then secured with the cohesive bandage to assist in focal compression over the treated vein. Then, 30 to 40 mm Hg compression stockings should be applied over the cohesive bandage. The optimal duration of compression following sclerotherapy is controversial and practice varies between 24 hours to 2 weeks. Compression is thought to improve treatment efficacy by reducing endoluminal caliber and thus thrombus volume, leading to more rapid vessel occlusion, with a lower risk of symptomatic thrombophlebitis and skin pigmentation. In addition, compression may reduce the incidence of DVT.[38] Patients should be advised to ambulate immediately following treatment to reduce risk of DVT and reduce reflux into the treated vein. To minimize venous distension, patients should be advised to avoid warm bath or sauna for 2 to 6 weeks following treatment. In addition, exercise resulting in an elevated intra-abdominal pressure such as running or weight lifting should be avoided for 1 to 2 weeks.[6,39]

Compression also has a role following sclerosant injection of reticular and telangiectatic veins and is believed to seal off the treated vein, reduce likelihood of recanalization, and minimize thrombophlebitis and hyperpigmentation.[37] In addition, placement of a small gauze pad or cotton wool ball directly over the injected vessel further increases local compression and minimizes bleeding. Although variations in practice exist, most physicians recommend compression of the sclerosed vessel with a 30 to 40 mm Hg graduated compression stocking for a minimum of 24 to 72 hours after treatment of leg telangiectasias.[40]

Sclerotherapy patients should be examined 2 weeks following treatment because it is not uncommon to see the development of symptomatic intravascular coagulum in larger treated vessels. This is often tender and may increase risk of hyperpigmentation. Accordingly, needle puncture and expression of the coagulated blood is advised.[41] Following administration of local anesthetic, a 19 G needle is introduced into the thrombosed vein and used to aspirate the coagulated blood, usually resulting in instant symptomatic relief.

Repeat treatment to the same area, if required, is not advised earlier than 6 to 8 weeks. This allows resolution of the sclerophlebitis to occur and also allows a better appreciation of the effectiveness of the prior treatment with a given solution and concentration.[6]

7.7 Complications of Sclerotherapy

When used appropriately, sclerotherapy is an effective treatment with a low incidence of complications.[42] However, side effects and complications associated with commonly used agents have been described and are discussed here.

7.7.1 Allergic and Drug Reactions

Anaphylactic shock following intravascular administration of sclerosing agents has been described but is exceedingly rare.[43] Nevertheless, the clinician should be on high alert in any patient with a history of multiple allergies and asthma. It is important that all clinicians using intravascular sclerosants have a well-established protocol for recognizing and treating severe allergic reactions, including rapid access to resuscitation equipment and medications including epinephrine, diphenhydramine, steroid, and supplemental oxygen.

At least six deaths have been reported with the use of STS, and its package insert recommends administration of a small test dose (0.5 mg) prior to full injection to observe for any allergic-type reactions.[18] Some authors, however, have attributed severe anaphylaxis to impurities within the sclerosant material (such as Carbitol) rather than the STS itself.[44] Less severe allergic reactions manifesting as hay fever and urticaria have an estimate incidence of 0.3% with STS.[44] An incidence of nonfatal allergies to POL of between 0.3 and 0.91% has been described.[44] In addition, two reports of fatal allergy following POL have been recorded.[6]

As mentioned briefly earlier, 1 mL of POL contains 40.5 mg of ethanol. As a result, patients taking the acetaldehyde dehydrogenase-inhibiting medication disulfiram (Antabuse; Wyeth-Ayerst Laboratories) have a theoretical risk of developing symptoms of the disulfiram reaction (headache, nausea, vomiting, flushing) following large-volume administration of intravenous POL.[45] This drug interaction remains hypothetical, however, as no such cases have been reported to date.[15]

7.7.2 Pain

STS is essentially painless when administered intravascularly but can cause pain when injected in the surrounding soft tissues. Some phlebologists have described reports of a dull ache within minutes following intravascular injection, which quickly resolves.[6] Given the anesthetic properties of POL, it does not produce pain when injected intravenously or in small quantities in the surrounding soft tissues. Studies comparing patient discomfort following intravascular STS and POL administration have shown no discernible difference.[46]

7.7.3 Tissue Necrosis

Local tissue necrosis may occur with extravasation of the sclerosant agent. The risk of skin necrosis rises with increasing volume and concentration. POL has a wide safety margin against skin necrosis caused by perivenous extravasation.[47] A study from Duffy et al involving the deliberate intradermal injection of POL and STS demonstrated that injection of 0.4 mL of 3% POL and 0.4 mL of 1% STS (doses of equal in vitro potency) resulted in tissue necrosis in the STS group only.[48]

Practitioners should be aware that extensive tissue necrosis can result from inadvertent intra-arterial injection of sclerosant agents, and the use of ultrasound guidance is advised for all nonvisible target veins. In the event of intra-arterial injection of sclerosant, consideration should be given to catheter-directed anticoagulation and thrombolysis.[49] Administration of systemic steroids may have a role in inflammation reduction.[50]

7.7.4 Pigmentation and Neovascularization (Matting)

Skin pigmentation following injection sclerotherapy has a highly variable frequency, with reports ranging from 0.3 to 30% in the short term.[51] Skin pigmentation tends to resolve slowly over weeks and months (▶ Fig. 7.5). As mentioned earlier, significant intravascular coagulum may be removed with needle puncture and expression to relief symptoms and reduce incidence of pigmentation. In addition, patients should be advised to avoid UV light exposure in the first 2 weeks following sclerotherapy.[2]

Matting (neovascularization) describes the new occurrence of fine telangiectasias in the area of a previously sclerosed vein. This phenomenon may also be seen following surgical treatment or thermal venous ablation. Adequate treatment of the underlying venous reflux is critical in avoiding this complication, which may also be exacerbated by initial high sclerosant concentration or volume. Rates of pigmentation and neovascularization with STS and POL are thought to be equivalent.[15]

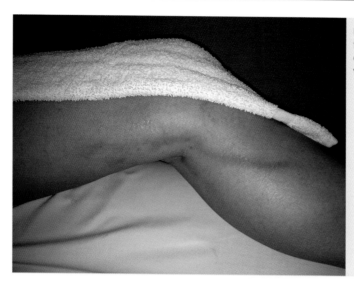

Fig. 7.5 Hyperpigmentation 3 months following 0.5% STS foam sclerotherapy of the distal GSV and associated calf varicosities.

7.7.5 Neurologic Events

Brief migraine-like symptoms have been described following liquid sclerotherapy but are more common following foam sclerotherapy.[52] Patients have described a scotoma with surrounding haziness or irregular colored patterns, which usually resolves within 30 minutes. Incidence varies significantly and has been reported to occur in as high as 2% of patients in some series.[33] However, a large registry of 6,395 foam injections described only 16 cases.[52] Such visual disturbances are believed to represent a migraine aura phenomenon rather than paradoxical gas or thromboembolism to the cerebral circulation.[53] Sclerosant-induced vasoconstrictor (endothelin 1 and serotonin) release are postulated mechanisms.[54,55] No demonstrable abnormalities have been observed at ophthalmic examination and no long-term visual defects have been reported.[2]

Since 1994, there have been 14 reported cases of stroke following sclerotherapy: 4 cases followed liquid sclerosant administration and a further 10 followed foam detergent sclerosant treatment. The most consistent risk factor among these patients was the presence of a right-to-left shunt and in particular a patent foramen ovale, suggesting either paradoxical gas or thromboembolism.[56] It should be remembered, however, that with a patent foramen ovale prevalence of 30% in the general population, the vast majority of patients with this condition have no neurologic sequelae following sclerotherapy.

Avoidance of large-volume injections of foam, avoidance of Valsalva maneuver in the early period following injection, and keeping the patient recumbent for a longer period of time may help reduce the incidence of neurologic symptoms.[2] In addition, all described cases of postsclerotherapy stroke have involved the use of room air in foam generation. To date, stroke has not been reported following the use of CO_2 in foam generation, and all neurologic events following its use have been transient. This may simply reflect that carbon dioxide is less commonly used in foam generation; however, further evaluation is warranted.

7.7.6 Thrombotic Complications

Severe thromboembolic events (proximal DVT and pulmonary embolus) are rare after sclerotherapy. The same large registry mentioned earlier reported one case of DVT after 12,173 sessions.[53] In a meta-analysis from Jia et al, the frequency of the DVT was 0.6%, the majority being distal in location.[24] The use of foam sclerosant in larger volumes, however, does increase the risk of thromboembolic complications especially when used in the treatment of truncal varices.[35] Generalized prothrombotic risk factors such as obesity, immobility, and use of medication such as oral contraceptive pills should be taken into account when calculating thromboembolic risk. As outlined earlier, careful technique including injecting "little and often," early application of 30 to 40 mm Hg compression stockings, periodic ankle dorsiflexion, and early ambulation all reduce risk of thrombotic complications.

7.8 New Techniques

New techniques involving the use of sclerosant agents such as mechanochemical ablation (MOCA) and industry-generated microfoam are discussed in detail in Chapter 10.

References

[1] Weiss RA, Feied CF, Weiss MA. Vein Diagnosis and Treatment: A Comprehensive Approach. New York, NY: McGraw Hill Medical Publishing; 2001

[2] Rabe E, Breu F, Cavezzi A, et al. Guideline Group. European guidelines for sclerotherapy in chronic venous disorders. Phlebology. 2014; 29(6):338–354

[3] Bradbury AW, Bate G, Pang K, Darvall KA, Adam DJ. Ultrasound-guided foam sclerotherapy is a safe and clinically effective treatment for superficial venous reflux. J Vasc Surg. 2010; 52(4):939–945

[4] Rasmussen LH, Lawaetz M, Bjoern L, Vennits B, Blemings A, Eklof B. Randomized clinical trial comparing endovenous laser ablation, radiofrequency ablation, foam sclerotherapy and surgical stripping for great saphenous varicose veins. Br J Surg. 2011; 98(8):1079–1087

[5] Ouvry P, Allaert FA, Desnos P, Hamel-Desnos C. Efficacy of polidocanol versus liquid in sclerotherapy of the great saphenous vein: a multicentrerandomised controlled trial with a 2-year follow-up. Eur J Vasc Endovasc Surg. 2008; 36 (3):366–370

[6] Goldman MP, Geux JJ, Weiss RA, eds. Sclerotherapy: Treatment of Varicose and Telangiectatic Leg Veins. 5th ed. Philadelphia, PA: Saunders Elsevier; 2011

[7] Lipton A, Harvey HA, Hamilton RW. Venous thrombosis as a side effect of tamoxifen treatment. Cancer Treat Rep. 1984; 68(6):887–889

[8] Breu FX, Guggenbichler S, Wollmann JC. 2nd European Consensus Meeting on Foam Sclerotherapy 2006, Tegernsee, Germany. Vasa. 2008; 37(71) Suppl 71:1–29

[9] Haudenschild CC, Schwartz SM. Endothelial regeneration. II. Restitution of endothelial continuity. Lab Invest. 1979; 41 (5):407–418

[10] Kobayashi S, Crooks S, Eckmann DM. Dose- and time-dependent liquid sclerosant effects on endothelial cell death. DermatolSurg. 2006; 32(12):1444–1452

[11] Chleir F, Vin F. Sclérus versus thrombus. Actua Vasc Inter. 1995; 35:18

[12] Dastain JY. Sclerotherapy of varices when the patient is on anticoagulants, with reference to 2 patients on anticoagulants. Phlebologie. 1981; 34:73

[13] Kanter AH. Complications of sotradecol sclerotherapy with and without heparin. In: Raymond-Martimbeau P, Prescott R, Zummo M, eds. Phlébologie '92. Paris: John Libbey Eurotext; 1992

[14] Mauriello J, Zygmunt J Jr. Synergistic effect of sclerosing agents. Eighth Annual Meeting of the North American Society of Phlebology. February 22, 1994

[15] Duffy DM. Sclerosants: a comparative review. DermatolSurg. 2010; 36(2) Suppl 2:1010–1025

[16] Imhoff E, Stemmer R. Classification and mechanism of action of sclerosingagents [in French]. Phlebologie. 1969; 22 (2):145–148

[17] STD Pharmaceutical Products Ltd. Prescribing Information. March 2012

[18] Sotradecol Product Insert, Bioniche Pharma Group Ltd, Revised March 2006

[19] Sadick N. Manual of Sclerotherapy. New York, NY: Lippincott Williams & Wilkins; 2000

[20] Cabrera Garido JR, Cabrera Garcia Olmedo JR, Garcia Olmedo D. Nuevo metodo de esclerosisen las varices tronculares. Patologia Vasculares. 1995; 1:55–72

[21] Orbach EJ, Petretti AK. The thrombogenic property of foam of a synthetic anionic detergent (sodium tetradecyl sulfate N.N. R.). Angiology. 1950; 1(3):237–243

[22] Foote RR. Varicose Veins. London: Butterworth& Co.; 1949

[23] Tessari L, Cavezzi A, Frullini A. Preliminary experience with a newsclerosing foam in the treatment of varicose veins. Dermatol Surg. 2001; 27(1):58–60

[24] Jia X, Mowatt G, Burr JM, Cassar K, Cook J, Fraser C. Systematic review of foam sclerotherapy for varicose veins. Br J Surg. 2007; 94(8):925–936

[25] Morrison N, Neuhardt DL, Rogers CR, et al. Comparisons of side effects using air and carbon dioxide foam for endovenous chemical ablation. J Vasc Surg. 2008; 47(4):830–836

[26] Beckitt T, Elstone A, Ashley S. Air versus physiological gas for ultrasound guided foam sclerotherapy treatment of varicose veins. Eur J Vasc Endovasc Surg. 2011; 42(1):115–119

[27] Alderman DB. Therapy for essential cutaneous telangiectasia. Postgrad Med. 1977; 61(1):91–95

[28] Mantse L. A mild sclerosing agent for telangiectasias. J Dermatol Surg Oncol. 1985; 11(9):855

[29] Leach BC, Goldman MP. Comparative trial between sodium tetradecyl sulfate and glycerin in the treatment of telangiectatic leg veins. Dermatol Surg. 2003; 29(6):612–614, discussion 615

[30] Jausion H. Glycerinechroméeetsclerose des ectasiesveineuses. Presse Med. 1933; 53:1061

[31] Duffy DM. Small vessel sclerotherapy: an overview. Adv Dermatol. 1988; 3:221–242

[32] Marley W. Low dose sotradecol for small vessel sclerotherapy. Newsl North Am Soc Phlebol. 1989; 3:3

[33] Coleridge Smith P. Sclerotherapy and foam sclerotherapy for varicose veins. Phlebology. 2009; 24(6):260–269

[34] de Roos KP, Groen L, Leenders AC. Foam sclerotherapy: investigating the need for sterile air. Dermatol Surg. 2011; 37 (8):1119–1124

[35] Myers KA, Jolley D. Factors affecting the risk of deep venous occlusion after ultrasound-guided sclerotherapy for varicose veins. Eur J Vasc Endovasc Surg. 2008; 36(5):602–605

[36] Leslie-Mazwi TM, Avery LL, Sims JR. Intra-arterial air thrombogenesis after cerebral air embolism complicating lower extremity sclerotherapy. Neurocrit Care. 2009; 11(1):97–100

[37] Kern P, Ramelet AA, Wütschert R, Hayoz D. Compression after sclerotherapy for telangiectasias and reticular leg veins: a randomized controlled study. J Vasc Surg. 2007; 45(6):1212–1216

[38] Villavicencio L. Handbook of Venous Disorders. London: Chapman and Hall Medical; 1996

[39] Stegall HF. Muscle pumping in the dependent leg. Circ Res. 1966; 19:180–190

[40] Weiss RA, Sadick NS, Goldman MP, Weiss MA. Post-sclerotherapy compression: controlled comparative study of duration of compression and its effects on clinical outcome. Dermatol Surg. 1999; 25(2):105–108

[41] Scultetus AH, Villavicencio JL, Kao TC, et al. Microthrombectomy reduces postsclerotherapy pigmentation: multicenter randomized trial. J Vasc Surg. 2003; 38(5):896–903

[42] Rathbun S, Norris A, Stoner J. Efficacy and safety of endovenous foam sclerotherapy: meta-analysis for treatment of venous disorders. Phlebology. 2012; 27(3):105–117

[43] Feied CF, Jackson JJ, Bren TS, et al. Allergic reactions to polido-canol for vein sclerosis. Two case reports. J Dermatol Surg Oncol. 1994; 20(7):466–468

[44] Nouri K. Complications in Dermatologic Surgery. St. Louis, MO: Mosby/Elsevier; 2008

[45] Williams SH. Medications for treating alcohol dependence. Am Fam Physician. 2005; 72(9):1775–1780

[46] Rao J, Wildemore JK, Goldman MP. Double-blind prospective comparative trial between foamed and liquid polidocanol and sodium tetradecyl sulfate in the treatment of varicose and telangiectatic leg veins. Dermatol Surg. 2005; 31(6):631–635, discussion 635

[47] Schuller-Petrović S, Pavlović MD, Neuhold N, Brunner F, Wöl-kart G. Subcutaneous injection of liquid and foamed polido-canol: extravasation is not responsible for skin necrosis during reticular and spider vein sclerotherapy. J Eur Acad Dermatol Venereol. 2011; 25(8):983–986

[48] Duffy DM, Hsu JTS, Alam M, Nguyen TH, eds. Procedures in Cosmetic Dermatology Series. the Netherlands: Elsevier; 2006; 71–106

[49] Grommes J, Franzen EL, Binnebösel M, et al. Inadvertent arte-rial injection using catheter-assisted sclerotherapy resulting in amputation. Dermatol Surg. 2011; 37(4):536–538

[50] Cavezzi A, Parsi K. Complications of foam sclerotherapy. Phlebology. 2012; 27 Suppl 1:46–51

[51] Goldman MP, Sadick NS, Weiss RA. Cutaneous necrosis, telan-giectatic matting, and hyperpigmentation following sclero-therapy. Etiology, prevention, and treatment. Dermatol Surg. 1995; 21(1):19–29, quiz 31–32

[52] Guex JJ, Allaert F-A, Gillet J-L, Chleir F. Immediate and mid-term complications of sclerotherapy: report of a prospective multicenter registry of 12,173 sclerotherapy sessions. Der-matol Surg. 2005; 31(2):123–128, discussion 128

[53] Gillet JL, Donnet A, Lausecker M, Guedes JM, Guex JJ, Leh-mann P. Pathophysiology of visual disturbances occurring after foam sclerotherapy. Phlebology. 2010; 25(5):261–266

[54] Frullini A, Di Stefano R. Endothelin release after sclerother-apy. International Symposium of Phlebology. Associazione Flebologica Italiana, Bologna, Italy 2007:2

[55] Agosti RM. 5HT1F- and 5HT7-receptor agonists for the treat-ment of migraines. CNS Neurol Disord Drug Targets. 2007; 6 (4):235–237

[56] Parsi K. Paradoxical embolism, stroke and sclerotherapy. Phlebology. 2012; 27(4):147–167

8 Ambulatory Phlebectomy

Indravadan J. Patel and Suvranu Ganguli

8.1 Introduction

Hippocrates is credited with performing the first phlebotomy to treat a varix circa 400 BC.[1] However, the surgical treatment of varicose veins was first described in detail by Aulus Cornelius Celsus (25 BC to 50 CE) in his medical text entitled *De Medicina*, which has been available since at least the Roman times. Through modification of technique and refinement of the available surgical tools, Swiss dermatologist Robert Muller reinvented the technique around 1956, and he has been referred to as "the father of modern day ambulatory phlebectomy."[2] Since the introduction of Muller's technique, there has been a natural evolution of ambulatory phlebectomy (AP), but the core principles in providing an efficient, minimally invasive, and economical procedure for varicose veins still hold true.

AP is a minor, outpatient surgical technique that removes dilated superficial varicose veins. The procedure is typically conducted on an ambulatory basis in all except the most severe cases. With the aid of local anesthesia, multiple microincisions allow for the complete removal of incompetent veins by hook avulsion, resulting in long-term success rates greater than 90%.[3,4] The procedure is generally well tolerated and complications are rare. Microsurgical phlebectomy, microphlebectomy, stab avulsion, and microextraction are synonymous with AP.

Exclusively performed with local anesthesia, AP leads to reduced surgical risks compared with traditional surgical venous ligation. The latter of the two leads to relatively high recurrence rates given that the vein is interrupted rather than removed.[5,6] Venous ligation has therefore fallen out of favor. In comparison, the problematic vein(s) is/are extracted with AP. The small size of the skin incision or puncture usually results in little or no scarring, typically producing good cosmetic results. AP may also be performed in conjunction with endovenous thermal ablation (EVTA) to provide the best available care in appropriately selected patients.

8.2 Indications

The main indication for AP is symptomatic varicose veins not responding to conservative treatment options such as compression therapy.

Superficial varicose veins near the skin surface are often too large to treat with sclerotherapy and too tortuous to treat with EVTA, making AP the optimal approach. AP may be used for the cosmetic aspect of treating asymptomatic varicose veins to treating complications of varices, such as recurrent superficial thrombophlebitis and bleeding.[7,8] AP for the treatment of small segments of superficial thrombophlebitis is readily performed. AP is effective in this setting as the involved vein segment as well as the intravascular coagulum can be extracted through the same incision. With experience, AP need not be exclusive to lower extremity varicose veins and is successfully performed on facial veins such as small periorbital or temporal veins.[9] Alternative indications for AP include vein biopsy and drug implant extraction.[10,11]

AP in the lower extremities permits removal of primary or secondary branch incompetent varicosities of the great saphenous vein (GSV) or small saphenous vein (SSV). The major tributary branch vessels of the GSV or SSV to be removed may include the anterior thigh circumflex vein, the posterior thigh circumflex vein, or anterior accessory GSV, particularly if they exhibit marked tortuosity. Additional varicose veins appropriate for AP include pudendal and labial veins of the groin. Perforators and dilated reticular veins may also be addressed.[12,13]

Dilated reticular veins around and below the knee, lateral thigh and leg, ankle, and venous network about the dorsum of the foot are less common indications for AP. Small reticular veins supplying or associated with telangiectasias, particularly about the foot and ankle, are less frequent indications for AP, but can be performed with success. A retrospective review of 75 patients who underwent AP of the foot demonstrated satisfactory results with few complications[14] (▶ Table 8.1).

With experience, foam sclerotherapy (Chapter 7) can satisfactorily treat large tortuous varicosities of the lower extremities, similar to AP. A determining factor in performing AP versus foam sclerotherapy for some practitioners includes assessment of the overall thickness of the venous wall. Thin-walled veins are typically better treated with foam sclerotherapy, whereas thicker-walled veins are generally reserved for AP.[15] Recurrence of varicose veins is significantly lower with AP when compared with sclerotherapy, as evidenced

Table 8.1 Indication and contraindication of AP

Indications	Contraindictions	
	Absolute	**Relative**
Asymptomatic varicose and reticular veins	Infectious dermatitis or cellulitis of area to be treated	Deep venous thrombosis
Symptomatic varicose and reticular veins	Severe peripheral edema	Nonambulatory patient
Complications of varicose veins	Seriously ill patients	Hypercoagulable state
	Severe allergy to local anesthetic	Anticoagulated patient
		Liver dysfuncton
		Pregnant or nursing

by a randomized controlled trial for the treatment of lateral accessory varicose veins comparing these two techniques. Two-year follow-up demonstrated a 2.1% recurrence rate with AP versus 37.5% for sclerotherapy.[16] Thrombophlebitis is also more common following sclerotherapy than AP.

Veins that may not be appropriate for AP include the GSV and SSV themselves as well as the saphenofemoral and saphenopopliteal junctions. These larger, deeper venous structures are below the superficial fascia and should not be addressed by AP. In such cases, EVTA with either radiofrequency or laser energy is indicated. It is quite commonplace to treat reflux of the saphenous system with EVTA, followed by AP of the remaining varicose branches in the same setting or at a follow-up procedure.

8.3 Contraindications

AP is contraindicated in cases of infectious dermatitis or cellulitis involving the area to be treated, as well as in severe peripheral edema or lymphedema. Patients who are seriously ill (e.g., severe cardiovascular or pulmonary problems), very elderly, or are unable to follow postoperative instructions should not be treated with AP. Patients on anticoagulation, uncorrectable coagulopathy, or hypercoagulable states pose a relative contraindication to AP. Other relative contraindications include patients who rely on the superficial venous system for drainage due to an occlusion of their deep venous system. Patients who are not able to ambulate postprocedure or those with severe peripheral arterial disease, preventing them from wearing compression stockings, are also not ideal candidates. An allergy to local anesthesia or

compromised liver function limiting the metabolism of the local anesthetic may pose relative contraindications. As tolerated, pregnant or nursing patients should have care of their varicose veins delayed to a later date (▶ Table 8.1).

8.4 Technique

8.4.1 Preprocedure

Procedure facilities, whether in a hospital or clinic setting, should have good lighting, a procedural table permitting Trendelenburg's position, and resuscitation equipment. Although allergic and toxic reactions are exceedingly rare, appropriate resuscitation capabilities should be available including intravenous fluid, epinephrine, diazepam, antihistamines, injectable steroids, and an automatic external defibrillator. A nurse or assistant should be present but direct intraoperative support is seldom necessary.

With the patient in the standing position, all varicose veins to be treated with AP should be identified, as it may be difficult or near impossible once in the recumbent position. A surgical permanent marker should be used to avoid washing away of the identifying marks during preparation of the site (▶ Fig. 8.1). Care should be taken during time of actual incision to avoid the marked areas, as a permanent tattoo may develop if the incisions were placed directly through the markings. Transillumination may also be used to accurately locate the vein(s) to be treated, enabling their removal with an overall reduction in size and number of incisions, as well as a decrease in operating time.[17,18]

Generally, premedication should be avoided and is rarely indicated because the best means of

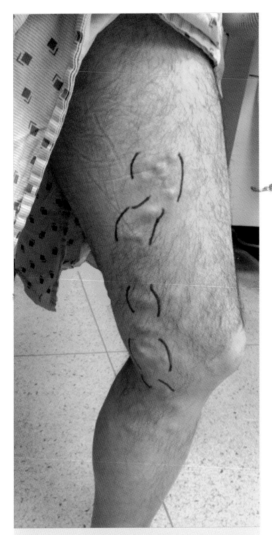

Fig. 8.1 All varicose veins are marked with the patient in the standing position given that they may be difficult or impossible to identify during recumbency. A permanent surgical marking is placed adjacent to the varicose vein to prevent washing away during preparation of the surgical site and to avoid accidently making an incision directly over the varicose vein itself. The microincisions should also not be made directly over the markings to avoid tattooing.

the addition of epinephrine. Epinephrine, at a concentration of 1:1,000,000, is frequently added to the solution because it slows down the absorption of lidocaine and it causes vasoconstriction of the superficial skin capillaries, minimizing postoperative bleeding. However, potential risks of adding epinephrine include tachycardia and skin necrosis. The addition of a buffer such as sodium bicarbonate to the acidic tumescent solution may neutralize the pH, making the infiltration less painful. The solution can be infused locally, using a series of large syringes, a pressurized bag, or a peristaltic pump. The use of tumescent anesthesia decreases patient discomfort during and after the procedure, and can contribute to predissection of the vein from the surrounding tissue, thereby elevating it to the skin surface and allowing for easier hook extraction.[21]

The procedure requires only a few surgical instruments. An 18-gauge cutting needle, an 11 blade scalpel, or a 15-degree ophthalmic blade may be used for the microincisions. Varying by size and shape, there are several commercially available vein hooks. The commonly used Muller's hooks of today are in fact an evolution of the broken half of a hemostat.[2] The modern-day Muller's hook is a blunt-tipped instrument resembling a crochet hook. The Oesch's hook is designed with a small barb at the tip, and is characterized by a large square handle, available in three sizes. The Ramelet's hook has a small fine hook with a distinct cylindrical shaft, also available in two sizes. Several other hooks serving a similar purpose include the Dortu, Varady, Vergereau, Martimbeau, and Trauchessec. Multiple clamps are required for AP. These clamps help maintain a firm grip on the extracted vein and should have fine serrated tips. Mosquito forceps can also be used to grasp veins as they are extracted. Surgical scissors and a spatula should readily be available.

8.4.2 Intraoperative

After the patient is placed on the procedural table, with the area to be treated prepped in a sterile fashion, tumescent anesthesia is injected into the perivenous tissue with care in avoiding the preprocedure markings. Cutaneous microincisions or punctures are made near the superficial varicose veins adjacent to the skin markings. The microincisions should be vertically oriented along the thigh, lower leg, and foot, while around the knee or ankle the incision should follow normal Langer's tension lines for a better cosmetic result. Care should be

preventing potential vascular complications is postoperative walking. Postoperative walking could be hindered in patients taking sedatives or anxiolytics.[19] Commonly, a large volume of low-concentration lidocaine known as tumescent anesthesia[20] should be instilled around the vein. Mixture concentrations range from 0.01 to 0.1% of lidocaine, at a dose of 4 mg/kg up to 7 mg/kg with

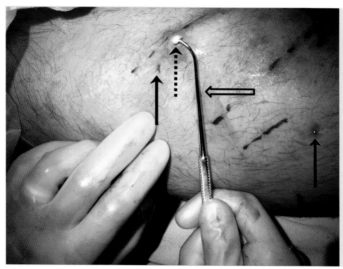

Fig. 8.2 Through the microincision (solid arrow), the phlebectomy hook (open arrow) is inserted along the course of the varicose vein (dashed arrow). After gentle dissection, the hook is rotated in a perpendicular direction. Once free, the vein can be brought out of the microincision with the hook. Note the size of the microincisions, approximately 1 to 3 mm in length, and the distance of the microincisions from the marked areas to avoid tattooing.

taken around the popliteal fold, the prepatellar, and pretibial region, as well as about the dorsum of the foot. These regions contain veins that may be more difficult to avulse and are therefore more susceptible to injury, such as a superficial hematoma about the popliteal fold.[22] The incisions themselves vary between 1 and 3 mm in size and can be separated from one another by 2 to 15 cm, dependent on the size and length of the vein, presence of perforators, and experience of the proceduralist.

Once the microincision has been made, the hook is inserted with the intention of undermining the varicose vein along its course via gentle dissection. The hook should then move in a perpendicular direction and rotated against the index vein. If there is difficulty in removing the vein from its perivenous fibroadipose attachments, a blunt dissector or spatula may be used. Once free, the vein can be brought out of the microincision with the hook (▶ Fig. 8.2). The liberated vein should then be grasped with either mosquito forceps or clamps outside of the microincision (▶ Fig. 8.3). Gentle traction on the vein allows the operator to remove short segments and may permit visualization of its entire course. Periodically, the clamps should be repositioned as the avulsed segments get longer and longer. At any time, the vein may be grasped between two clamps and cut with surgical scissors to facilitate removal. Through repetition, the entire varicose vein or a segment of it is progressively extracted from one microincision to the next. Hemostasis is achieved during the procedure by applying light compression with sterile gauze.

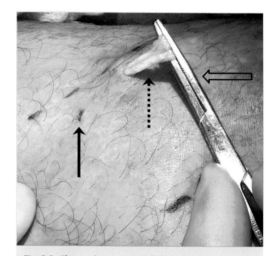

Fig. 8.3 Clamps (open arrow) help maintain a firm grip on the extracted vein (dashed arrow) and should have a fine serrated tip. The vein is grasped outside of the microincision (solid arrow) with clamps. Multiple clamps and repositioning of the clamps closer to the microincision site can be used to avulse longer segments.

In general, aggressive hooking should be eliminated to minimize complications. If the patient experiences pain while attempting removal of the vein, a nerve may accidently be hooked. Alternatively, if the vein requires an increased amount of tension for removal, a tendon could mistakenly be hooked. However, an attempt at removal of all parts of the varicose vein should be made to reduce the possibility of superficial thrombophlebitis of a retained segment.

Only after significant experience should AP around the knee, pretibial area, ankle, and foot be undertaken. These regions are more susceptible to injury as previously mentioned. Risk of superficial hematomas and sensory nerve injury is increased.[22,23] AP behind the knee should be done with care given that the skin is thin and friable, increasing the likelihood of enlarging microincisions by overzealous hooking. AP of the foot should be performed in the dorsiflexed position to minimize complications.

8.4.3 Postoperative

Skin closure is not necessary if the microincisions or puncture sites are kept to 1 to 3 mm in size. Leaving the microincision open allows for drainage of the tumescent anesthetic fluid, improving cosmetic results. If oozing is persistent, this may easily be controlled with light compression or with elevation of the leg. The leg should then be cleaned, followed by placement of sterile gauze, gauze wrap, or pads covering the microincisions. Care should be taken to avoid antiseptic powder or solution because it may induce silicotic granulomas,[24] nor should tape or adhesive bandages be applied directly to the microincisions given that it may increase the risk of allergic dermatitis and blistering.

A highly elastic bandage is then applied to the leg to achieve compression of the treated area. The bandage is applied distally, beginning at the foot and terminating proximally, covering all incisions. The compression dressing reduces postprocedure complications, including pain, hemorrhage, bruising, and seroma formation. The dressing should be performed by someone with experience to avoid a tourniquet effect. Use of a class II closed-toe graduated compression stocking (30–40 mm Hg) over the elastic bandage dressing is recommended for additive compression.[16]

A trial walk should occur after the elastic bandage and compression stockings have been secured to ensure patient comfort and to check for signs of any immediate complications such as bleeding. Walking helps to minimize postprocedural complications and is crucial in the healing process. Following AP, patients are encouraged to ambulate and return to activities of daily living, with the caveat that they should not participate in strenuous lower extremity aerobic exercises for at least 2 weeks to avoid increased pressure within the treated area. Driving an automobile may be delayed by at least 24 hours because the tumescent anesthesia may result in a subtle transient impairment on distal motor function. Likewise, prolonged periods of immobility, such as with bed rest or travel, should be avoided to decrease the risk of deep venous thrombosis.

Reported pain levels are low following AP and easily controlled with over-the-counter medications such as ibuprofen or acetaminophen. If more pain control is required, the proceduralist may provide a prescription for acetaminophen with codeine (Tylenol #3) or acetaminophen with oxycodone (Percocet), as tolerated.

8.5 Follow-up

The dressing and stockings should be left intact immediately following the procedure, and then taken off for showering after the second or third postoperative day. It is recommended that the compression stockings then be worn during the day only for a total of 1 to 4 weeks following this initial visit. The amount of compression therapy depends on the degree of reflux treated, the size and number of varicose veins removed, and the amount of residual bruising. Early skin exposure to sunlight may result in hyperpigmentation and should be avoided for a better cosmetic outcome. The patient should return to the office 7 to 14 days after the procedure, dependent on the clinician and the extent of area treated. The microincisions should be checked for proper healing and the dressings should be discontinued at this time. Follow-up appointments should be made at approximately 4 to 12 weeks, 6 months, and 1 year. These subsequent visits are necessary to document and treat any complications, ensure overall success of the procedure, and to assess the need for additional intervention.

Most complications secondary to AP are minor and benign and resolve spontaneously over time. The causes may be anesthetic related, poor technique, or secondary to postprocedure dressing and care. Complications may be classified as cutaneous, vascular, lymphatic, or neurologic. Major complications of AP are exceedingly rare and generally AP is considered a safe procedure. A variety of complications and the reported rates of such complications within the literature are presented in ▶ Table 8.2, a modification of the Standards of Practice multidisciplinary quality improvement guideline for the treatment of lower extremity superficial venous insufficiency with AP put forth by the Society of Interventional Radiology, Cardiovascular Interventional

Table 8.2 Complications of AP

	Common	Rate	Rare	Rate
Cutaneous	Blister formation	4 to 6%	Contact dermatitis	<0.1 to 1%
	Transient pigmentation	3 to 6%	Keloid formation	
	Telangiectactic matting	2 to 4%	Tatooing	
			Infection	
			Foreign body granuloma	
Vascular	Superficial thrombophle-bitis (localized)	2 to 3%	Delayed bleeding	<0.1 to 0.1%
	Hermatoma	<1 to 1%	Deep venous thrombosis/pul-monary embolism	
			Superficial thrombophlebitis (extensive)	
Lymphatic			Lymphocele	<0.1 to 0.5%
			Persistent edema	
Neurologic			Dysesthesia	<0.1 to 0.5%
			Carpotarsal syndrome	
			Traumatic neuroma	
Anesthetic			Allergic reaction	<0.1 to 0.1%
			Technique related	

Radiological Society of Europe, and the American College of Phlebology.[8,22]

At the 1- to 3-month postoperative visit, the need for additional intervention is assessed. If small residual reticular veins or telangiectasias persist, complementary sclerotherapy may be indicated. If many large varicose veins are present, the source of the venous reflux may not have been adequately treated by AP. In such cases, GSV or SSV reflux should be addressed with EVTA techniques or sclerotherapy. EVTA with AP is fast, effective, and safe with complete remission of patient-reported leg pain and fatigue at up to 2 years post-treatment.[25] The benefits of combined EVTA plus AP include improvement in quality-of-life scores and decrease in number of additional procedures.[26,27] Concomitant treatment strategies are a sound approach given that AP may be performed concurrently or posttreatment of proximal venous reflux. This combined stepwise approach may allow the varicosities to decrease in size and even normalize downstream of the treated area, obviating the need for AP altogether.

When AP is performed in the appropriate patient, or complementary to an alternative therapy, the long-term results are excellent.[3,4] However, certain areas of the body, including the foot, the hands, and the area around the eyes, are notably more difficult to treat by AP.[23] Although the varicose veins are physically extracted from the body, removing the diseased veins at any one time does not prevent the development of new varices over the years. This is dependent on a multitude of factors such as familial/genetic or may be related to one's personal history such as occupation, lack of physical activity, body weight, or pregnancy status. For these reasons, patients must be regularly followed up for the possible progression and development of varicose veins and venous insufficiency over time.

References

[1] Olivencia JA. History of the surgical treatment of varicose veins of the lower extremities. J Phlebol. 2001; 1:11–16

[2] Olivencia JA. Ambulatory phlebectomy turned 2400 years old. Dermatol Surg. 2004; 30(5):704–708, discussion 708

[3] Ramelet AA. Phlebectomy. Technique, indications and complications. Int Angiol. 2002; 21(2) Suppl 1:46–51

[4] Olivencia JA. Minimally invasive vein surgery: ambulatory phlebectomy. Tech Vasc Interv Radiol. 2003; 6(3):121–124

[5] Critchley G, Handa A, Maw A, Harvey A, Harvey MR, Corbett CR. Complications of varicose vein surgery. Ann R Coll Surg Engl. 1997; 79(2):105–110

[6] Ramelet AA. La phlébectomie ambulatoire selon Muller: technique, avantages, désavantages. J Mal Vasc. 1991; 16 (2):119–122

[7] Oesch A. Indications for and results of ambulatory varices therapy [in German]. Ther Umsch. 1991; 48(10):692–696

[8] Kundu S, Grassi CJ, Khilnani NM, et al. Cardiovascular Interventional Radiological Society of Europe, American College of Phlebology, and Society of Interventional Radiology Standards of Practice Committees. Multi-disciplinary quality improvement guidelines for the treatment of lower extremity superficial venous insufficiency with ambulatory phlebectomy from the Society of Interventional Radiology, Cardiovascular Interventional Radiological Society of Europe, American College of Phlebology and Canadian Interventional Radiology Association. J Vasc Interv Radiol. 2010; 21(1):1–13

[9] Weiss RA, Ramelet AA. Removal of blue periocular lower eyelid veins by ambulatory phlebectomy. Dermatol Surg. 2002; 28(1):43–45

[10] De Roos KP, Neumann HA. Vein biopsy. A new indication for Muller's phlebectomy. Dermatol Surg. 1995; 21(7):632–634

[11] Lam M, Tope WD. Surgical pearl: phlebectomy hook Norplant extraction. J Am Acad Dermatol. 1997; 37(5, Pt 1):778–779

[12] Ramelet AA. Phlebectomy—cosmetic indications. J Cosmet Dermatol. 2002; 1(1):13–19

[13] Ramelet AA, Perrin M, Kern P, Bounameaux H. Phlebology. 5th ed. Paris: Elsevier Science; 2008

[14] Olivencia JA. Ambulatory phlebectomy of the foot. Review of 75 patients. Dermatol Surg. 1997; 23(4):279–280

[15] Weiss RA, Dover JS. Leg vein management: sclerotherapy, ambulatory phlebectomy, and laser surgery. Semin Cutan Med Surg. 2002; 21(1):76–103

[16] de Roos KP, Nieman FH, Neumann HAM. Ambulatory phlebectomy versus compression sclerotherapy: results of a randomized controlled trial. Dermatol Surg. 2003; 29 (3):221–226

[17] Weiss RA, Goldman MP. Transillumination mapping prior to ambulatory phlebectomy. Dermatol Surg. 1998; 24(4):447–450

[18] Spitz GA, Braxton JM, Bergan JJ, et al. Outpatient varicose vein surgery with transilluminated powered phlebectomy. Vasc Surg. 2000; 34:547–555

[19] Cohn MS, Seiger E, Goldman S. Ambulatory phlebectomy using the tumescent technique for local anesthesia. Dermatol Surg. 1995; 21(4):315–318

[20] Klein JA. Anesthesia for liposuction in dermatologic surgery. J Dermatol Surg Oncol. 1988; 14(10):1124–1132

[21] Smith SR, Goldman MP. Tumescent anesthesia in ambulatory phlebectomy. Dermatol Surg. 1998; 24(4):453–456

[22] Olivencia JA. Complications of ambulatory phlebectomy: A review of 4000 consecutive cases. Am J Cosmet Surg. 2000; 17:161–165

[23] Ricci S, Georgiev M, Goldman MP, et al. Phlebectomy. In: Ricci S, Georgiev M, Goldman MP, eds. Ambulatory Phlebectomy. New York, NY: Taylor & Francis Group; 2005:135–144

[24] Ramelet AA. An unusual complication of ambulatory phlebectomy. Talc granuloma [in French]. Phlebologie. 1991; 44 (4):865–871

[25] Goldman MP, Amiry S. Closure of the greater saphenous vein with endoluminal radiofrequency thermal heating of the vein wall in combination with ambulatory phlebectomy: 50 patients with more than 6-month follow-up. Dermatol Surg. 2002; 28(1):29–31

[26] Carradice D, Mekako AI, Hatfield J, Chetter IC. Randomized clinical trial of concomitant or sequential phlebectomy after endovenous laser therapy for varicose veins. Br J Surg. 2009; 96(4):369–375

[27] Fernández CF, Roizental M, Carvallo J. Combined endovenous laser therapy and microphlebectomy in the treatment of varicose veins: Efficacy and complications of a large single-center experience. J Vasc Surg. 2008; 48(4):947–952

9 Safety, Quality, and Complications

Ann L. Brown, Lauren Ferrara, and Felipe B. Collares

9.1 Introduction

Adverse events and complications related to interventional procedures can still occur despite the best efforts of the phlebologists. The culture of safety in health care has been extensively promoted and patient safety regulations and guidelines by specialty societies have been implemented to increase safety and improve quality. Hospitals have made substantial investments in patient safety and quality assurance in recognition of a number of complications related to surgical care. Surgical safety checklists were designed to incorporate safety protocols, minimize information loss, and promote efficient communication in the operating room. These same principles apply to phlebology procedures performed in the hospital setting or in the outpatient office.

The number of phlebology interventions performed, as well as the complexity and variety of these procedures, has increased significantly in the recent years. Despite the fact that hospitals have the infrastructure and expertise to address complications and emergencies, the office setting has become appealing to phlebologists and patients due to its convenience and cost effectiveness. Compared to hospitals, the office setting can be more pleasant to patients, usually offers improved access in convenient locations, and has lower operational costs. On the other hand, hospitals can offer prompt emergency support, electronic access to medical records and imaging, and availability of different medical specialties, which are lacking in the office setting.

In order to explore all the advantages of the office setting, and at the same time provide safe outpatient procedures, phlebology clinics should implement safety practices similar to the inpatient setting. The culture of safety in the office setting should include all aspects of patient care, from the initial contact with the patient to the assessment of posttreatment satisfaction.

A detailed medical history should be obtained and a physical examination with ultrasound evaluation of the lower extremity venous system should be performed. Pertinent information must be recorded and documented, which may include digital photographs of visible veins in the legs. The office setting should offer adequate space for staff circulation in the procedure room and light sources for the physical and ultrasound examinations. All members of the team involved with patient care should know the availability and location of emergency equipment, the protocols for cardiopulmonary emergencies, the protocols for emergency transfer of patients, and the fire evacuation protocol. For easy consult, written emergency protocols may be displayed in the procedure room.

Immediate preprocedure measures should include the following:
- Review of the patient's medical history and essential imaging studies.
- Written informed consent explaining the risks, benefits, and alternatives to the procedure.
- Confirmation of the patient identity and the procedure to be performed.
- Adequate identification of site and side of the procedure.
- Confirmation that postprocedure materials are available for immediate use, such as compression dressing or stocking.

Before discharging the patient, the following measures are recommended:
- Assessment for pain and immediate postprocedure complications, such as bleeding and deep venous thrombosis (DVT).
- Adequate cleaning and dressing of the treated area.
- Patient education with detailed postprocedure instructions—written instructions are preferable and can be offered with contact phone numbers.
- Plan for postdischarge follow-up.

9.2 Risk Assessment and Prevention in the Phlebology Clinic

9.2.1 Awareness and Understanding of Deep Venous Thrombosis

DVT poses a challenge to physicians and is a major health problem. Every physician involved with phlebology is well aware of the risks and potential consequences of DVT. Virchow's triad of hypercoagulability, venous stasis, and endothelial injury highlight the pathophysiologic causes of DVT. Patients presenting for venous interventions often have many conditions and habits that increase their risk for the development of DVT, which are usually the same factors that led to the need for venous intervention.

Risk factors for DVT, although well known, merit repeating and should be investigated in every patient during their preoperative visit and physical examination. The risk factors include the following: history of a previous DVT; recent surgery or trauma; immobilization; malignancy; coagulopathies, either acquired or inherited—including factor V Leiden mutation; prothrombin gene mutation; antithrombin III deficiency; protein C and protein S deficiencies; antiphospholipid antibody syndrome; hyperhomocysteinemia; and plasma hyperviscosity states. The risk of DVT is also increased in pregnancy, in the postpartum state, and in patients on hormone therapy. To a lesser extent, the risk of DVT is elevated in patients with congestive heart failure, inflammatory bowel disease, obesity, and advanced age. Primary valvular insufficiency was also described as a minor risk factor for DVT. Although the risk of DVT is smaller in patients with these comorbidities than the aforementioned risk factors, the risk during venous interventions may be additive or perhaps exponentially increased due to the risks inherent to the procedure.[1,2]

Patients should be carefully screened if there is a family history of DVT or known family history of a thrombophilia. Not only are the pathologic causes of thrombosis often present in patients presenting with venous insufficiency, but also these pathologic factors are altered during each venous intervention:

- Sclerosant agents entering the vein likely cause a transient hypercoagulable state.
- A significant number of patients requiring venous interventions are sedentary. Pain following the procedure may further contribute to decreased activity, which leads to venous stasis.
- Interventional procedures cause endothelial injury and occlusion of the superficial vein; however, untargeted endothelial injury or thrombus extension may lead to DVT.

The combination of preexisting risk factors and risk factors associated with the procedure compound the risk of DVT.[1,2]

9.2.2 Can Venous Intervention Be Performed in Patients with a History of DVT?

Venous interventions can be performed and are frequently requested for patients with a history of DVT; however, the risk of recurrence should be investigated. Stratification of the risk of recurrence can be assessed as follows:

- "Provoked" DVT: It includes patients whose DVT occurred due to temporary or reversible risk factors including long-distance flight, surgery, or major trauma. The risk of recurrence is considered low.
- "Unprovoked"/idiopathic DVT: It includes patients with known malignancies or coagulation disorders, or patients in whom no etiology is identified. The risk of recurrence is considered high.

The presence of residual thrombus after anticoagulation therapy also increases the risk of recurrence. Accordingly, patients who may have been initially classified in the "provoked"/low-risk group but presented with residual thrombus on a 6-month follow-up ultrasound are considered high risk. Furthermore, the risk of recurrence is higher in patients with proximal (iliofemoral) DVT in comparison with distal (femoropopliteal) DVT.[3,4]

9.2.3 To Treat or Not to Treat: Deciding to Treat or to Postpone Therapy

The myriad of DVT risk factors among patients and the variations in the severity (and the patients perception of the severity) of the varicose vein disease render the development of official guidelines a difficult and challenging task, which is why there is very little guidance in the current literature.

The decision to treat or defer therapy should take in consideration the risks and benefits of the intervention. The severity of patients' symptoms and potential improvement following venous intervention should be carefully assessed on an individual basis, with attention to risk factors and the risk of recurrent DVT in particular.

Most physicians would consider deferring therapy if the patient has had recent major surgery, major trauma, immobilization, or pregnancy. Other conditions in which avoidance of venous interventions should be considered include patients with cancer, thrombophilia, and idiopathic DVT, unless significant improvement in the quality of life would result.

9.2.4 Preventive Measures in Patients with High Risk of DVT in Whom Venous Therapy Is Deemed Appropriate

- *Steps to prevent DVT*. It is well known that early ambulation and mechanical or pharmacologic prophylaxis prevent DVT. The importance and necessity of early ambulation should be emphasized at length regardless of the anticipated risk of DVT. Patients should receive compression therapy, most commonly compression stocking in the postoperative period, and be educated about the importance of early and continued ambulation as well as continued compliance with compression therapy.
- *Awareness of DVT*. Patients should be educated about the common symptoms of DVT both prior to scheduling the procedure and on the day of the procedure. This may also be available in the written postprocedure instructions provided to patients and include contact information to reach the clinical staff if symptoms occur.
- *Pharmacologic prophylaxis in high-risk patients*. To date, there are no convincing data to support the routine use of anticoagulation prophylaxis for venous interventions such as endovenous thermal ablation or sclerotherapy. In theory, patients with hypercoagulable states may benefit from periprocedural anticoagulation; however, there is no consensus protocol for drug of choice, timing, or duration of anticoagulation.[5] Although not commonly done, some phlebologists recommend a short course of 3 to 5 days of subcutaneous administration of low-molecular-weight heparin (LMWH) in high-risk patients such as patients with cancer, thrombophilia, or idiopathic DVT.[2]
- *Technique of venous therapy*. Diligence and sound technique in theory should prevent DVT for many reasons. During endovenous thermal ablation, the tip of the delivery catheter should always be visualized to prevent activation in an undesired location causing untargeted endothelial injury. Some authors propose the use of liquid sclerosants rather than foam for high-risk patients given that foam produces greater endothelial injury and an increased transient iatrogenic hypercoagulable state. Extensive interventions performed in one setting may increase significantly the length of the procedure and recovery time. Two or more separate procedure sessions should be considered for high-risk cases to limit the time the patient is sedentary. It is a well-established practice to encourage ambulation after venous interventions because long periods of immobility could increase the risk of DVT.[2]

9.3 Complications of Phlebology Interventions

Venous thromboembolic complications can result from different phlebology interventions and possibly represent the major concern during the postprocedure follow-up.

9.3.1 Superficial Thrombophlebitis

Superficial thrombophlebitis (ST) is a common inflammatory process associated with thrombosis of a superficial vein. Clinical signs and symptoms include localized pain, erythema, pruritus, edema, tenderness, and hardening of the surrounding tissue. Although there is some evidence to suggest an association between ST and venous thromboembolism,[6] further investigation is needed to clarify the correlation between ST and DVT.

In the literature, controversy exists over the definition of ST after sclerotherapy. Sclerotherapy of varicose veins induces a desired inflammatory reaction that will eventually evolve into fibrosis. Therefore, inflammation including erythema, pain, tenderness, edema, and hardening of the vein at the site of venous injection should not be interpreted as phlebitis. Consensus defines ST as superficial venous thrombosis in a noninjected vein. However, the difference between ST and an excessive but expected sclerotherapy reaction could be difficult to distinguish.

ST occurs after sclerotherapy and its incidence in the literature ranges from 0 to 46% with a mean of 5%[7,8,9,10,11]; however, the real frequency of ST as defined above is unknown.

There is no difference in the rate of ST for foam compared to liquid sclerosants. However, the relative risk of ST is increased for foam sclerotherapy when compared with laser therapy and surgery.[8]

Prevention

Early ambulation and the use of graduated compression stockings are thought to be important to decrease the development of ST in dependent tributary veins, although this is not based on data.

Anecdotally, ST is more commonly associated with large-diameter-dependent varicose veins or varicose tributaries following occlusion of their inflow and outflow. Therefore, concurrent phlebectomy of such veins can be performed at the time of endovenous therapy to prevent ST.[5]

Treatment

Treatment aims to improve and relieve local painful symptoms but also to prevent additional thromboembolic events, which could complicate the natural course of ST. ST has been managed in most series with nonsteroidal anti-inflammatory drugs (NSAIDs), graduated compression stockings, and ambulation. However, one large placebo-controlled randomized, controlled trial of 3,002 patients showed a significant reduction in symptomatic superficial venous thrombosis in patients treated with prophylactic fondaparinux for 6 weeks.[12]

The evidence on oral treatments, topical treatment, or surgery is too limited to inform clinical practice.[13] Further research is needed on the novel oral anticoagulants (NOACs) including direct thrombin and activated factor X inhibitors, LMWH, and NSAIDs to evaluate the effect on superficial venous thrombosis and ST progression, and to determine optimal doses and durations of therapy or combination therapies.

9.3.2 Deep Venous Thrombosis

DVT of the lower extremities following phlebology interventional procedures is considered a major complication since it can be associated with substantial morbidity. The development of pulmonary embolism can be life threatening. The late manifestation of postthrombotic syndrome (PTS) is also being recognized as the end-stage sequela of inadequately treated DVT. Permanently painful and swollen legs, pigmentation, skin deterioration, and venous ulceration in severe cases characterize this syndrome. In the absence of effective therapy, PTS patients have a reduced quality of life.[14]

Few studies are available to evaluate the real frequency of DVT occurring after liquid sclerotherapy given that most published studies on liquid sclerosant are old and predate routine duplex ultrasound (DUS). The incidence of DVT is reportedly low in studies utilizing foam sclerosant, ranging from less than 1% to 1.8%.[8,15,16,17,18] The occurrence

of DVT after endovenous thermal ablation of a superficial vein is uncommon, with reported incidences of 0.3% for laser ablation and 0.4% after radiofrequency ablation.[5]

Endovenous Heat-Induced Thrombosis

Endovenous heat-induced thrombosis (EHIT) is defined as extension of thrombus from the thermal-ablated superficial vein into the adjacent deep vein. It can be illustrated as propagation of thrombus from the great saphenous vein into the common femoral vein through the saphenofemoral junction or from the small saphenous vein into the popliteal vein through the saphenopopliteal junction (▶ Fig. 9.1). Classification of EHIT is based on the extent of thrombus propagation into the deep venous system as follows[19,20,21]:

- Class 1: Propagation of thrombus to the level of the junction between the superficial and deep venous systems.
- Class 2: Propagation of thrombus from the ablated superficial vein into the deep venous system with less than 50% intraluminal occlusion.
- Class 3: Propagation of thrombus from the ablated superficial vein into the deep venous system with more than 50% intraluminal occlusion.
- Class 4: Propagation of thrombus from the ablated superficial vein into the deep venous system with complete intraluminal occlusion.

Symptomatic and asymptomatic DVTs are not often distinguished in the literature, although there is a likely clinical significant difference in the outcome. Severe thromboembolic events such as proximal DVT, pulmonary embolism, or paradoxical embolization are very rare complications of phlebology interventions. Most cases of DVT diagnosed by DUS on routine follow-up are distal and asymptomatic.[7,16]

Prevention

Individual risk assessment for the development of venous thromboembolism for elective general surgery patients can be performed utilizing the Caprini risk assessment model.[22] The most recent American College of Chest Physicians (ACCP) guidelines include recommendations for DVT risk stratification with the Caprini score to determine the need for thromboprophylaxis in an individual

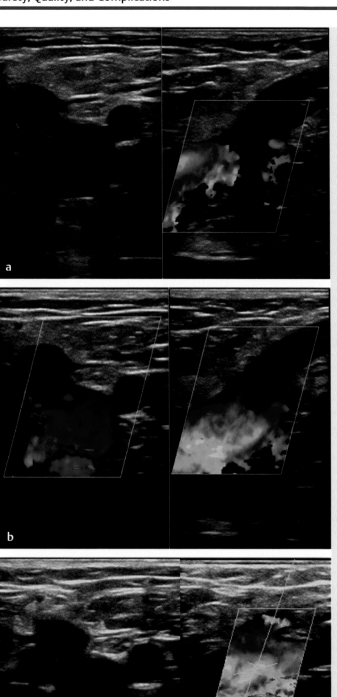

Fig. 9.1 A 55-year-old man with symptomatic varicose veins related to significant venous reflux in the left great saphenous vein (GSV). Medications in use include aspirin and Plavix indicated by the past medical history of coronary artery disease with stent placement. Endovenous laser ablation was performed without interruption of anticoagulation therapy. Immediate postprocedure ultrasound examination showed no evidence of DVT at the left common femoral vein (CFV). **(a)** One-week follow-up: axial and sagittal views of the left CFV at the level of the saphenofemoral junction (SFJ) showing propagation of thrombus with less than 50% occlusion—EHIT Class 2. **(b)** Twelve-day follow-up: axial and sagittal views of the left CFV at the level of the SFJ showing thrombus at the level of the SFJ—EHIT Class 1. **(c)** One-month follow-up: axial and sagittal views of the left CFV at the level of the SFJ showing thrombus in the proximal left GSV without involvement of the SFJ.

patient.[23] Thromboprophylaxis includes pharmacologic (heparin or enoxaparin) and physical (compression and ambulation) prophylaxis.

Increased risk of thrombosis is associated with the use of larger volumes of sclerosant, particularly in the form of foam.[10,24,25] Patients with a history of venous thromboembolism or thrombophilia are also at increased risk. Therefore, a careful risk–benefit assessment should be performed prior to treatment. Periprocedural anticoagulation may be considered; however, the indications for use, drug choice, duration of therapy, and efficacy of such prophylaxis have not been well studied. A randomized, controlled trial comparing a 10-day regimen of LMWH in combination with ambulation and compression therapy to ambulation and compression therapy alone showed no difference in a moderate-risk population.[26]

Following venous interventions such as endovenous thermal ablation and sclerotherapy, early ambulation and graduated compression stockings are recommended.[5,27] Patients should be counseled to avoid prolonged immobilization and long-distance travel in the first week after the procedure to reduce the risk of thromboembolic events. Compression stockings should also be worn daily in the postprocedure period, usually for 1 to 2 weeks,[5] but protocols may vary significantly between different institutions.

Diagnosis

Acute DVT refers to clinical symptoms present for less than 14 days or imaging findings indicating thrombosis within the last 14 days. Only half of patients present with classic symptoms of pain, swelling, and tenderness of the lower extremity.[28] Nevertheless, clinical history and physical examination are critical in the initial workup of any patient with suspected DVT.

The extent of disease is classified as proximal or distal. Proximal thrombosis may involve complete or partial occlusion of the inferior vena cava and/or the iliac, common femoral, deep femoral, femoral, and/or popliteal veins. Proximal thrombosis should be more precisely characterized as iliofemoral or femoropopliteal based on the involved venous segments.[29] Distal thrombosis involves complete or partial occlusion of the deep calf veins including the anterior tibial, posterior tibial, peroneal, and/or deep muscular veins.

The diagnosis and extent of DVT can be established on imaging with DUS or venography performed indirectly on computed tomography (CT) or magnetic resonance imaging (MRI), or directly by interventional radiology. DUS is typically the first and most frequently used imaging modality. To date, neither CT nor MRI has been validated for DVT diagnosis. The hallmark finding on DUS is noncompressibility of the thrombosed vein.

Institutional protocols for DUS may vary but should involve interrogation of all proximal veins with compression at a minimum according to the ACR and AIUM guidelines (American College of Radiology and American Institute of Ultrasound in Medicine). ICAVL (Intersocietal Commission for the Accreditation of Vascular Laboratories) guidelines suggest additional interrogation of the posterior tibial and peroneal veins of the calf. As a caveat, both sets of guidelines stipulate additional evaluation of symptomatic areas if the cause of symptoms is not elucidated by the standard examination.[30]

Recent venous intervention increases the pretest probability of DVT. Additional risk factors should be taken into consideration when deciding whether to pursue diagnosis with imaging, especially in asymptomatic patients or patients with symptoms confined to the calf. The primary goal of diagnostic testing is to identify patients who will benefit from anticoagulant therapy. In the reformed 2012 ACCP guidelines, routine whole-leg ultrasound is disfavored over other approaches. For example, if an isolated distal DVT is suspected clinically, this does not need to be sought out or treated in the absence of severe symptoms. If proximal extension is a concern, a proximal ultrasound is recommended in 1 week to exclude the need for anticoagulation. Conversely, if risk is high, objective testing for DVT is indicated, even in the absence of symptoms given the unreliability of clinical assessment and the consequences of a missed diagnosis.[23]

Treatment

Current treatment strategies include systemic anticoagulation, surgical thrombectomy, and catheter-directed thrombolysis (CDT) with or without stent placement. Traditional systemic anticoagulation forms the basis of adequate treatment with effective prevention of thrombus extension, pulmonary embolism, death, and recurrence of DVT. Endovascular therapy (with thrombolysis, mechanical thrombectomy, and stent placement), however, can offer faster relief of symptoms and prevent PTS.[31,32,33,34,35]

Current ACCP guidelines for a provoked DVT (whether proximal or distal) are as follows[23]:

In the acute phase, an initial course of LMWH or fondaparinux is recommended over the use of unfractionated heparin. LMWH or fondaparinux should be administered once a day by subcutaneous injection to bridge a patient to a therapeutic dose of an oral anticoagulant. Oral anticoagulation should be started early and the bridge therapy should be continued for at least 5 days or until the international normalized ratio is 2.0 or above for at least 24 hours.

The options for oral anticoagulation are expanding. Vitamin K antagonists are the mainstay of treatment but NOACSs such as dabigatran etexilate (Pradaxa), rivaroxaban (Xarelto), apixaban (Eliquis), and edoxaben (Lixiana) are showing promise in large phase 3 trials. Rivaroxaban and dabigatran were shown to have comparable efficacy and bleeding risk.[36]

Long-term anticoagulation of a provoked DVT or an isolated DVT in the calf can be prescribed for a shorter duration than unprovoked DVT because the risk of recurrent DVT is low. Treatment for 3 months is recommended over longer durations of therapy, at which time the risk–benefit ratio should be reassessed.

Medical management of DVT does not seem to be influenced by surgical or radiologic interventions including stenting. Recent ACCP 2012 guidelines stipulate the same intensity and duration of anticoagulant therapy in patients who have undergone any method of thrombus removal.[23] In acute DVT, immediate anticoagulation is prudent to reduce the risk of recurrent thrombosis and extension of thrombus. Long-term anticoagulation therapy can be personally tailored based on a patient's common risk factors for recurrent thrombosis and individual risk of bleeding. Typical dosages for anticoagulants are listed in ▶ Table 9.1.

Early Thrombus Removal

Much data demonstrate that systemic anticoagulation alone does not protect against the common late sequela of DVT, PTS. With anticoagulation alone, the incidence of PTS is as high as 50 to 56% in patients with iliofemoral DVT.[31,32] Early thrombus removal techniques are being investigated to reduce the morbidity associated with PTS by restoring venous flow and preserving the function of venous valves. At least two techniques, surgical thrombectomy and CDT, have been shown to significantly reduce the risk of developing PTS compared to systemic anticoagulation in patients with

Table 9.1 Typical dosages for anticoagulants[23,26,29,30,31,36]

Low-molecular-weight heparin	
Enoxaparin	1 mg/kg twice a day or 1.5 mg/kg once a day
Dalteparin	200 units/kg (first 30 d)
	150 units/kg (maintenance)
Fondaparinux	
< 50 kg	5 mg/d
50 to 100 kg	7.5 mg/d
> 100 kg	10 mg/d
Direct thrombin and factor Xa inhibitors	
Rivaroxaban	15 mg twice a day for 3 wk for initial anticoagulation, followed by 20 mg once a day
Apixaban	10 mg twice a day for 7 d for initial anticoagulation, followed by 5 mg twice daily for 6 mo
Edoxaban	60 mg once a day
Dabigatran	150 mg twice daily
Warfarin	

Initial dose of 5 mg/d for the first 2 d (range: 2–10 mg/d). Dose is then adjusted until the international normalized ratio is within the therapeutic range (2–3; target 2.5)

iliofemoral DVT.[29,31] Currently, insufficient data limits comparison of surgical thrombectomy to CDT. Studies have demonstrated both techniques to be feasible, safe, and effective.[29,31,32,33]

Risk factors for developing PTS include proximal vein involvement (common femoral or iliac veins), extensive thrombus, prior ipsilateral thrombosis, obesity, advanced age, and female sex. There is insufficient evidence at present to support early thrombus removal in patients with isolated femoropopliteal DVT.[34]

In ambulatory patients with good functional capacity, the following strategies may be considered for early thrombus removal in the setting of acute iliofemoral DVT and are strongly recommended in the setting of limb-threatening ischemia due to iliofemoral venous obstruction[29]:

Surgical Thrombectomy

A variety of techniques can be employed to achieve thrombectomy. Most commonly, a catheter-mounted angioplasty balloon is used to remove gross or macroscopic fragments of thrombus from the iliac veins via an incision in the groin. Additional catheter-based mechanical devices are used to remove associated distal thrombus by microscopic fragmentation, maceration, and/or aspiration. Adjunctive construction of an arteriovenous fistula is recommended by some to reduce early rethrombosis.[29]

Catheter-Directed Thrombolysis

In CDT, thrombolytic agents are infused through a multiside hole catheter placed directly into a venous thrombus via a remote puncture site. Additional catheter-based mechanical devices are used to achieve thrombus fragmentation, diffusion of thrombolytics, and aspiration of thrombus. Regional thrombolysis results in more rapid dissolution of the thrombus as well as reduced bleeding complications when compared to systemic administration.[32]

The CaVenT study is the first multicenter prospective randomized, controlled trial to show the benefit of CDT. The study demonstrated an absolute risk reduction in the development of PTS for patients undergoing CDT without stenting in combination with anticoagulation compared to anticoagulation alone (41% compared to 56%).[32]

Venograms performed during CDT permit a detailed evaluation of the affected vein during and after endovenous thrombus removal. An underlying proximal venous stenosis has been reported in as many as 80% of patients with iliofemoral DVT.[35, 37] Addressing this underlying anatomic stenosis with adjunctive venous stenting and/or balloon angioplasty following CDT may be crucial to restore good venous outflow and prevent recurrence. This practice is widely used in the United States.[33] However, further research is necessary to evaluate whether CDT with stenting alone or in combination with anticoagulation is superior to any of the previously studied therapies.

Contraindications to Thrombolytic Therapy

Contraindications to thrombolytic therapy include the following[33]:
- Active internal bleeding.

- Recent cerebrovascular accident or intracranial surgery.
- Recent serious gastrointestinal bleeding.
- Major trauma or surgery (within 10 days).
- Severe uncontrolled hypertension.
- Pregnancy.
- Endocarditis.
- Intracardiac thrombus or known right-to-left shunt.
- Coagulopathy, thrombocytopenia, or absolute contraindication to anticoagulation.
- Suspected septic thrombus.
- Allergy to thrombolytic agents.

Associated risks of CDT include hemorrhage (particularly intracranial), pulmonary embolism, and recurrent DVT. Adverse events overall have been poorly reported in comparative trials. Some evidence of bleeding complications has been reported, most commonly involving the venous access site (4%) but also the retroperitoneum (1%).[29]

9.3.3 Other Complications and Risks

Complications related to phlebology interventions can range from mild pain or minor cosmetic complaints to serious adverse events. Fortunately, major complications related to phlebology procedures are rare, and most cases do not cause permanent injury or sequelae. Most common adverse events related to specific phlebology procedures were addressed in the respective chapters and noteworthy complications are summarized here.

Anaphylactic Shock

Anaphylactic shock as a result of allergic reaction to the sclerosant agent is regarded as an extremely rare complication but constitutes an emergency. If suspected, the injection should be halted immediately and the operator should proceed with standard life support including the administration of epinephrine when appropriate.[38]

Tissue Necrosis

Local tissue necrosis can occur with extravasation of sclerosant, and the risk increases in proportion with the volume and the concentration of the agent. Inadvertent intra-arterial injection of sclerosant

Table 9.2 Characteristics of different local anesthetic medications, including maximum recommended doses[40]

Agent	Relative potency	Onset time	Duration	Max. dose (mg)	Max. dose (mg/kg)
Chloroprocaine	4	Very quick	Short	600	10
Lidocaine	1	Quick	Medium	300	4–5
Mepivacaine	1	Quick	Medium	300	4–5
Ropivacaine	4	Slow	Long	200	2.5–3
Bupivacaine	4	Slow	Long	175	2.5
Tetracaine	16	Slow	Long	100	1.5

occurs rarely and may result in large tissue necrosis. If injection is associated with severe pain, the procedure should be halted immediately. If intra-arterial injection is suspected, CDT should be performed when possible. This may be coupled with systemic anticoagulation. Additionally, systemic steroid administration may reduce inflammation.[9]

Neurologic Complications

Neurologic complications related to sclerotherapy are rare and can vary from brief migraine-like symptoms and temporary visual disturbances to thromboembolic stroke. Transient symptoms can occur after liquid sclerotherapy but are more common with use of foam. Severe neurologic complications are extremely rare but are possible due to foam passage into the cerebral circulation through a right to left heart shunt.[39]

Local Anesthetic Adverse Reactions

Characteristics of different local anesthetic agents are listed in ▶ Table 9.2. Adverse reactions to local anesthetic are not rare; fortunately, however, most reactions are psychosomatic responses secondary to anxiety and stress. True allergic reactions are rare. Phlebology procedures such as phlebectomy and endovenous thermal ablation may require large volumes of tumescent anesthesia with very dilute anesthetic. Good injection technique with careful needle placement and ultrasound guidance should avoid intravascular delivery of significant amount of local anesthetic and the risk of overdose and toxicity. Systemic toxicity is directly related to the plasma concentration of the drug. Initial symptoms usually include tongue and perioral numbness, lightheadedness, involuntary muscle contraction, and eventually depressed level of consciousness and seizures. As serum levels of local anesthetic increase, respiratory depression and cardiovascular collapse may occur. Management of severe local anesthetic systemic toxicity includes the following[40,41]:

- Initiate the protocol of emergency transfer of the patient from the outpatient setting.
- Supplemental administration of oxygen.
- Administration of anticonvulsant such as a benzodiazepine (midazolam or diazepam) or barbiturate to raise seizure threshold or treat seizure activity.
- Advanced cardiac life support in cases of respiratory depression or cardiac collapse.

Cosmetic Complications

Most patients undergoing phlebology procedures are looking not only for symptomatic relief related to venous insufficiency but also for cosmetic improvement of their legs. In many cases, the cosmetic aspect is the major concern for patients consulting with a phlebologist. Cosmetic complications of venous interventions include bruising, blistering, scarring, skin pigmentation, and neovascularization and should be discussed with patients prior to the procedure and included in the informed consent. Pre- and postprocedure photographs are also crucial in the assessment of cosmetic improvement.

Good clinical and cosmetic outcomes depend on proper procedural technique and adequate postprocedure management. Patients should be educated to ensure compliance with postprocedure instructions regarding skin care, use of compression stocking, and avoidance of sun light exposure when appropriate. Furthermore, phlebologists should openly discuss cosmetic improvement with patients and encourage realistic expectations.

References

[1] Ten Cate-Hoek AJ, Prins MH, Wittens CHA, ten Cate H. Postintervention duration of anticoagulation in venous surgery. Phlebology. 2013; 28 Suppl 1:105–111

[2] Vedantham S. Superficial venous interventions: assessing the risk of DVT. Phlebology. 2008; 23(2):53–57

[3] Prandoni P, Lensing AW, Prins MH, et al. Residual venous thrombosis as a predictive factor of recurrent venous thromboembolism. Ann Intern Med. 2002; 137(12):955–960

[4] Douketis JD, Crowther MA, Foster GA, Ginsberg JS. Does the location of thrombosis determine the risk of disease recurrence in patients with proximal deep vein thrombosis? Am J Med. 2001; 110(7):515–519

[5] Khilnani NM, Grassi CJ, Kundu S, et al. Cardiovascular Interventional Radiological Society of Europe, American College of Phlebology, and Society of Interventional Radiology Standards of Practice Committees. Multi-society consensus quality improvement guidelines for the treatment of lower-extremity superficial venous insufficiency with endovenous thermal ablation from the Society of Interventional Radiology, Cardiovascular Interventional Radiological Society of Europe, American College of Phlebology and Canadian Interventional Radiology Association. J Vasc Interv Radiol. 2010; 21(1):14–31

[6] Decousus H, Quéré I, Presles E, et al. POST (Prospective Observational Superficial Thrombophlebitis) Study Group. Superficial venous thrombosis and venous thromboembolism: a large, prospective epidemiologic study. Ann Intern Med. 2010; 152(4):218–224

[7] Guex JJ, Allaert FA, Gillet JL, Cheir F. Immediate and midterm complications of sclerotherapy: report of a prospective multicenter registry of 12,173 sclerotherapy sessions. Dermatol Surg. 2005; 31(2):123–128, discussion 128

[8] Rathbun S, Norris A, Stoner J. Efficacy and safety of endovenous foam sclerotherapy: meta-analysis for treatment of venous disorders. Phlebology. 2012; 27(3):105–117

[9] Cavezzi A, Parsi K. Complications of foam sclerotherapy. Phlebology. 2012; 27 Suppl 1:46–51

[10] Myers KA, Jolley D. Factors affecting the risk of deep venous occlusion after ultrasound-guided sclerotherapy for varicose veins. Eur J Vasc Endovasc Surg. 2008; 36(5):602–605

[11] Min RJ, Khilnani N, Zimmet SE. Endovenous laser treatment of saphenous vein reflux: long-term results. J Vasc Interv Radiol. 2003; 14(8):991–996

[12] Decousus H, Prandoni P, Mismetti P, et al. CALISTO Study Group. Fondaparinux for the treatment of superficial-vein thrombosis in the legs. N Engl J Med. 2010; 363(13):1222–1232

[13] Di Nisio M, Wichers IM, Middeldorp S. Treatment for superficial thrombophlebitis of the leg. Cochrane Database Syst Rev. 2013; 4(4):CD004982

[14] Kahn SR, Hirsch A, Shrier I. Effect of postthrombotic syndrome on health-related quality of life after deep venous thrombosis. Arch Intern Med. 2002; 162(10):1144–1148

[15] Guex JJ. Complications of sclerotherapy: an update. Dermatol Surg. 2010; 36 Suppl 2:1056–1063

[16] Gillet JL, Guedes JM, Guex JJ, et al. Side-effects and complications of foam sclerotherapy of the great and small saphenous veins: a controlled multicentre prospective study including 1,025 patients. Phlebology. 2009; 24(3):131–138

[17] Bergan J, Pascarella L, Mekenas L. Venous disorders: treatment with sclerosant foam. J Cardiovasc Surg (Torino). 2006; 47(1):9–18

[18] Jia X, Mowatt G, Burr JM, Cassar K, Cook J, Fraser C. Systematic review of foam sclerotherapy for varicose veins. Br J Surg. 2007; 94(8):925–936

[19] Kabnick LS. Complications of endovenous therapies: statistics and treatment. Vascular. 2006; 14:S31–S32

[20] Dexter D, Kabnick L, Berland T, et al. Complications of endovenous lasers. Phlebology. 2012; 27 Suppl 1:40–45

[21] Anwar MA, Lane TR, Davies AH, Franklin IJ. Complications of radiofrequency ablation of varicose veins. Phlebology. 2012; 27 Suppl 1:34–39

[22] Caprini JA, Arcelus JI, Reyna JJ. Effective risk stratification of surgical and nonsurgical patients for venous thromboembolic disease. Semin Hematol. 2001; 38(2) Suppl 5:12–19

[23] Gould MK, Garcia DA, Wren SM, et al. American College of Chest Physicians. Prevention of VTE in nonorthopedic surgical patients: Antithrombotic Therapy and Prevention of Thrombosis, 9th ed: American College of Chest Physicians Evidence-Based Clinical Practice Guidelines. Chest. 2012; 141 (2) Suppl:e227S–e277S

[24] Forlee MV, Grouden M, Moore DJ, Shanik G. Stroke after varicose vein foam injection sclerotherapy. J Vasc Surg. 2006; 43 (1):162–164

[25] Breu FX, Guggenbichler S, Wollmann JC. 2nd European Consensus Meeting on Foam Sclerotherapy 2006, Tegernsee, Germany. Vasa. 2008; 37 Suppl 71:1–29

[26] San Norberto García EM, Merino B, Taylor JH, Vizcaíno I, Vaquero C. Low-molecular-weight heparin for prevention of venous thromboembolism after varicose vein surgery in moderate-risk patients: a randomized, controlled trial. Ann Vasc Surg. 2013; 27(7):940–946

[27] Rabe E, Breu F, Cavezzi A, et al. European guidelines for sclerotherapy in chronic venous disorders. Phlebology. 2014; 29 (6):338–354

[28] Bounameaux H, Perrier A, Righini M. Diagnosis of venous thromboembolism: an update. Vasc Med. 2010; 15(5):399–406

[29] Meissner MH, Gloviczki P, Comerota AJ, et al. Society for Vascular Surgery, American Venous Forum. Early thrombus removal strategies for acute deep venous thrombosis: clinical practice guidelines of the Society for Vascular Surgery and the American Venous Forum. J Vasc Surg. 2012; 55(5):1449–1462

[30] Tenna AM, Kappadath S, Stansby G. Diagnostic tests and strategies in venous thromboembolism. Phlebology. 2012; 27 Suppl 2:43–52

[31] Casey ET, Murad MH, Zumaeta-Garcia M, et al. Treatment of acute iliofemoral deep vein thrombosis. J Vasc Surg. 2012; 55 (5):1463–1473

[32] Enden T, Haig Y, Kløw NE, et al. CaVenT Study Group. Long-term outcome after additional catheter-directed thrombolysis versus standard treatment for acute iliofemoral deep vein thrombosis (the CaVenT study): a randomised controlled trial. Lancet. 2012; 379(9810):31–38

[33] Vedantham S, Thorpe PE, Cardella JF, et al. CIRSE and SIR Standards of Practice Committees. Quality improvement guidelines for the treatment of lower extremity deep vein thrombosis with use of endovascular thrombus removal. J Vasc Interv Radiol. 2009; 20(7) Suppl:S227–S239

[34] Kahn SR, Shrier I, Julian JA, et al. Determinants and time course of the postthrombotic syndrome after acute deep venous thrombosis. Ann Intern Med. 2008; 149(10):698–707

[35] Kwak HS, Han YM, Lee YS, Jin GY, Chung GH. Stents in common iliac vein obstruction with acute ipsilateral deep venous thrombosis: early and late results. J Vasc Interv Radiol. 2005; 16(6):815–822

[36] Ahrens I, Peter K, Lip GY, Bode C. Development and clinical applications of novel oral anticoagulants. Part I. Clinically approved drugs. Discov Med. 2012; 13(73):433–443

[37] Chung JW, Yoon CJ, Jung SI, et al. Acute iliofemoral deep vein thrombosis: evaluation of underlying anatomic abnormalities by spiral CT venography. J Vasc Interv Radiol. 2004; 15 (3):249–256

[38] Feied CF, Jackson JJ, Bren TS, et al. Allergic reactions to polidocanol for vein sclerosis. Two case reports. J Dermatol Surg Oncol. 1994; 20(7):466–468

[39] Parsi K. Paradoxical embolism, stroke and sclerotherapy. Phlebology. 2012; 27(4):147–167

[40] Culp WC, Jr, Culp WC. Practical application of local anesthetics. J Vasc Interv Radiol. 2011; 22(2):111–118, quiz 119

[41] Hatsiopoulou O, Cohen RI, Lang EV. Postprocedure pain management of interventional radiology patients. J Vasc Interv Radiol. 2003; 14(11):1373–1385

10 New Endovascular Techniques

Edward H. Ahn and Felipe B. Collares

10.1 Introduction

Endovenous thermal ablation for refluxing great saphenous veins (GSVs) has become increasingly common in practice over the past decades and has proven safe and effective,[1,2,3] replacing traditional ligation or stripping in several societal guidelines[4] as first-line therapy. Thermal ablative techniques include both laser and radiofrequency (RF) devices, previously discussed in detail in Chapter 6.

Thermal ablation methods require tumescent anesthesia, which provides several benefits, including compressive vein wall apposition to allow more efficient ablation, local anesthesia to avoid systemic sedation, and a heat sink to protect adjacent soft tissue from thermal injury. Nonetheless, despite its essential role for thermal ablation, administration of tumescent anesthesia adds to procedure time and has been shown to be more painful than the ablation procedure itself.[5] Additionally, there is also a small associated risk of lidocaine toxicity.[6] It should also be noted that postprocedural care for both laser and RF ablation includes the utilization of compression stockings, which itself can be a source of discomfort.

Though thermal ablation is highly effective and time-proven, there has been strong interest in the development of nonthermal ablative techniques as these obviate the need for tumescent anesthesia, since there is no heating of soft tissues, therefore potentially decreasing procedure time and procedure-associated pain. Nonthermal ablation also circumvents potential side effects intrinsic to thermal ablation including sensory nerve damage and bruising.

This chapter will detail the three nonthermal techniques with the greatest substance of science and literature behind them, including polidocanol (POL) endovenous microfoam sclerotherapy (Varithena), mechanochemical ablation (MOCA; ClariVein), and cyanoacrylate embolization (CAE; VenaSeal). Additional nonthermal techniques described at the end of the chapter are currently considered more experimental, with less published evidence.

10.2 Endovenous Microfoam Sclerotherapy/Varithena

10.2.1 Overview

Foam sclerotherapy refers to administration of a liquid sclerosant that has been mixed with gas to produce a foam preparation. While foam can be manually compounded via the Tessari technique (Chapter 7), Varithena is a pharmaceutical grade, low-density, injectable POL microfoam that is formulated via a proprietary canister system. Currently, in the United States, Varithena is the only Food and Drug Administration (FDA)–approved foam for treatment of incompetent GSVs. In the proprietary Varithena formulation, POL, the sclerosant agent, is mixed with oxygen, carbon dioxide, and an ultra-low amount of nitrogen within a canister to produce a 1% POL microfoam solution.[7,8,9,10,11,12,13,14,15]

Absolute contraindications for foam sclerotherapy include severe allergy to the sclerosant, acute deep vein thrombosis (DVT) or pulmonary embolism, local infection in the limb to be treated, and long-lasting immobility. The procedure should be avoided in pregnant and nursing patients. Relative contraindications for foam sclerotherapy include severe peripheral arterial disease, high thromboembolic risk, and superficial thrombophlebitis.[16,17]

10.2.2 Mechanism of Action

The mechanism of action of sclerosant agents is discussed in detail in Chapter 7. In summary, the POL foam displaces blood instead of mixing with it, maximizing endothelial surface contact area and time. POL disrupts the osmotic barrier of the venous endothelium, leading to vessel wall damage and vasospasm. As a result, the interior surface of the vein becomes thrombogenic, leading to thrombosis and occlusion. The occluded vein is eventually replaced by fibrous connective tissue.[7,8,9,10]

As compared to manually compounded foam, the Varithena foam has been found to have smaller and more homogeneous bubble size (▶ Fig. 10.1). The median bubble diameter of Varithena is less

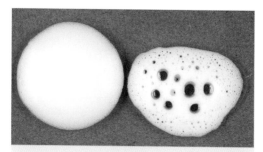

Fig. 10.1 Varithena foam (left) compared to manually compounded foam (right). (Reproduced with permission from BTG.)

than 100 µm and no bubbles are greater than 500 µm. Compared to physician-compounded foam, the Varithena foam has a slower degradation rate in ex-vivo models, which may correlate to increased vein contact time.[11]

10.2.3 Varithena® Device and Technique

The Varithena® device holds two sterile, connected, 303-mL aluminum alloy canisters: one contains POL solution, 180 mg/18 mL (10 mg/mL), under a carbon dioxide atmosphere, and the second contains pressurized oxygen at approximately 5.4 bar absolute. The connector joins the two canisters allowing activation of the product (▶ Fig. 10.2). Once activated, Varithena injectable foam delivers a 1% POL solution, and each mL of Varithena injectable foam contains 1.3 mg of POL. One canister of Varithena generates a total volume of 90 mL of foam, which is sufficient to yield 45 mL of usable foam for intravenous injection. Once activated, the Varithena canister must be used within 7 days.[16]

The vein to be treated is accessed via a micropuncture set or equivalent using aseptic technique under ultrasound guidance. The vein should be accessed distally. For example, when treating GSV insufficiency, the vessel is punctured near the level of the knee. The micropuncture sheath can be used for treatment or exchanged for an appropriately sized catheter (16–22 gauge). A manometer tubing (supplied with the Varithena kit) is prefilled with heparinized normal saline and then connected to the catheter. With the tube and catheter secure, the leg is elevated to 45 degrees. The Varithena canister is then activated to generate foam and then a transfer unit is attached to the canister (▶ Fig. 10.3). Up to 5 mL of foam at a time are transferred to a syringe. No visible air bubbles

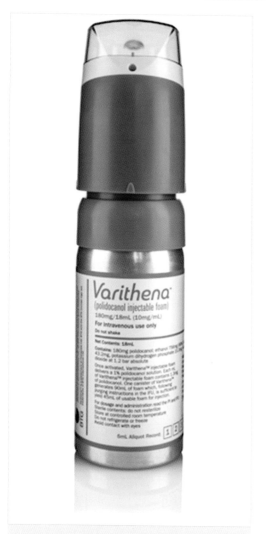

Fig. 10.2 Varithena canister with transfer unit attached. (Reproduced with permission from BTG.)

should be seen within the foam. Once extracted into the syringe, the foam must be administered within 75 seconds.[16]

The syringe of freshly generated foam is connected to the manometer tubing. Foam is injected slowly under ultrasound monitoring and continued until the foam reaches a point 3 to 5 cm distal to the saphenofemoral junction (SFJ). Long catheters may also be used to precisely deposit foam throughout the vein.[18,19] Additional foam may be injected distally to fill the distal GSV and major varicose tributaries. Venospasm of treated veins is confirmed via ultrasound, with some authors advocating manual compression on the SFJ during foam administration to minimize flow of foam into

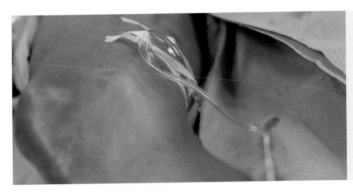

Fig. 10.3 Manometer tubing filled with Varithena foam, attached to intravenous catheter. (Reproduced with permission from BTG.)

the femoral vein.[20] The recommended injection rate is approximately 1 mL/second in the GSV and 0.5 mL/second in accessory varicosities. A new sterile syringe is used after each injection. Up to 5 mL of foam may be used per injection and no more than 15 mL should be used per treatment session. Compression stockings with compression pads should be immediately applied and be worn for at least 2 weeks after treatment to assist with vein closure.[16]

10.2.4 Outcomes

Literature suggests that manually compounded, nonproprietary foam sclerotherapy is less effective than thermal ablation of truncal incompetent veins. A meta-analysis evaluating 64 studies for anatomic success, defined as obliteration or disappearance of treated veins, demonstrated 3-year success rates of 95% for endovenous laser ablation, 84% for RF ablation, and 77% for foam sclerotherapy.[21]

The VANISH-2 study[8] compared Varithena versus placebo in patients with SFJ incompetence due to reflux of the GSV or major accessory veins. Clinical improvement in symptoms of varicose veins at week 8 after treatment (as measured via a VVSymQ score) was seen in 80.5% of the pooled Varithena group (which included both 0.5 and 1.0% POL formulations) versus 21.2% of the placebo group. Duplex ultrasound response (defined as either elimination of SFJ reflux and/or complete occlusion of the incompetent vein seen at baseline) was seen in 85.6% of the pooled Varithena group versus 1.8% of the placebo group.[8]

Results after treatment with Varithena were also found to be durable with ongoing improvement. Of the 56 patients followed to 1 year after treatment, 77.2% had improved symptoms at 8 weeks and 86.0% at 1 year. Similarly, 70.2% of patients reported improved appearance at 8 weeks and 87.7% at 1 year.[10]

10.2.5 Complications

In Varithena placebo-controlled trials,[7,8] the most common postprocedure adverse reaction with the Varithena was pain in the treated extremity (15%), along with limb discomfort (7–12%) and pain at the injection site (7–10%). A total of 80% of pain episodes in the treated limb resolved within 1 week. Additional adverse reactions included superficial thrombophlebitis (5–9%), nonocclusive thrombus extending from the superficial vein into the common femoral vein (2.9%), proximal DVT (1.7%), and distal DVT (1.1%). Contusion or hematoma of the injection site was seen in 9% of patients. There were no reported events of nerve damage. Hyperpigmentation of the treated limb was noted in 1.1% of patients treated with Varithena.

In the VANISH-2 trial[8] using Varithena foam, there were no clinically significant neurologic or visual adverse events. Cerebral gas embolism, however, has been found to be of concern when physician-compounding methods are used to create foams. The incidence of neurologic or visual adverse events with those preparations is approximately 2% and is predominantly transient.[11,13] Complications related to foam sclerotherapy are discussed in detail in Chapters 7 and 9.

10.3 Mechanochemical Ablation/ClariVein®

10.3.1 Overview

MOCA refers to a hybrid method of endovenous ablation utilizing both mechanical abrasion via a rotating wire tip and simultaneous chemical ablation via injection of liquid sclerosant, either sodium tetradecyl sulfate (STS) or POL. The MOCA device (▶ Fig. 10.4) was developed in 2005 and is currently marketed under the tradename ClariVein®. Contraindications for MOCA are similar to

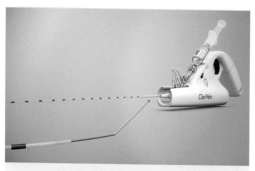

Fig. 10.4 The ClariVein device and wire tip. (Reproduced with permission from Vascular Insights, LLC.)

those of sclerotherapy procedures discussed in Chapter 7 and include allergic reaction to the sclerosant agent, acute DVT or pulmonary embolism, local infection of the limb to be treated, peripheral arterial disease, and pregnancy.[22,23,24,25,26,27,28,29,30,31,32]

10.3.2 Mechanism of Action

The MOCA technique combines mechanical damage to the endothelium caused by the rotating wire with the chemical damage caused by the infused sclerosant agent. The mechanical damage promotes coagulation activation by damaging the endothelium; induces local vasospasm and decreases the diameter of the treated vein; promotes better distribution of the sclerosant within the vascular lumen; and increases the action of the sclerosant agent by mechanical damage to the endothelium (▶ Fig. 10.5). The liquid sclerosant further damages the lipid cell membrane of the endothelium, ultimately resulting in occlusion and fibrosis of the treated vein.[22] Liquid rather than foam sclerosant is advised by the manufacturer for this hybrid technique due to lack of FDA approval for intravascular use of manually compounded foams as well as possible side effects and complications seen with foam administration. Histologic analysis of a GSV 1 year after MOCA demonstrated circumferential disappearance of the endothelium and fibrosis of the vein. The media was also considerably damaged with collagen changes.[22]

10.3.3 ClariVein® Device and Technique

The ClariVein® device is composed of two components, an infusion catheter and a battery motorized handle. A syringe containing the liquid

sclerosant (STS or POL) attaches to the handle. The catheter (45 or 65 cm in length with an outer diameter of 0.035 inches) contains a rotating wire that is activated and controlled by the handle. A small metal ball is attached to the angled tip of the wire (▶ Fig. 10.6). The diameter of rotation of the wire tip is 6.5 mm, but the effective diameter is larger due to wire oscillation during rotation.

At the beginning of the procedure, a micropuncture or equivalent intravascular access is obtained distally into the vessel to be treated under ultrasound guidance and after administration of local anesthesia. The ClariVein catheter, detached to the handle, is then advanced through the vascular access to the desired proximal ablation edge under direct ultrasound guidance. For ablation of the GSV, the tip of the wire should be positioned 2 cm distal to the SFJ. For small saphenous vein (SSV) ablation, the wire tip should be positioned within the initial portion of the superficial straight segment of the SSV distal to the saphenopopliteal junction. No tumescent anesthesia or patient sedation is required.[22,23,24,25,26,27,28]

After appropriate positioning under ultrasound guidance, the catheter is attached to the device handle. Once the catheter and handle are attached, they cannot be disassembled. The sclerosant syringe is attached to the handle, and then the tip of the wire is unsheathed under ultrasound guidance, ensuring no proximal migration. When the handle is gripped with one hand, the index finger can activate the trigger for the motor and the thumb is used to depress the sclerosant syringe plunger. The maximum motor rotation speed, 3,500 rpm, is the default speed and is the most often used.[22,23,24,25,26,27]

Wire rotation without administration of sclerosant agent is recommended initially for 3 seconds to induce venospasm at the proximal segment of the treated vessel, followed by continued spinning and pullback with infusion of sclerosant. The recommended pullback speed is between 1 and 2 mm/second.[24,28] Similar results have been obtained with the use of STS or POL as the sclerosant agent. The total volume of sclerosant is based on the diameter and length of the vein and is usually 6 to 10 mL for GSV and 2 to 4 mL for SSV treatment.[28] Compression stockings are recommended for 2 weeks after MOCA.

10.3.4 Outcomes

The MOCA procedure has been demonstrated to be less painful than RF ablation for treatment of

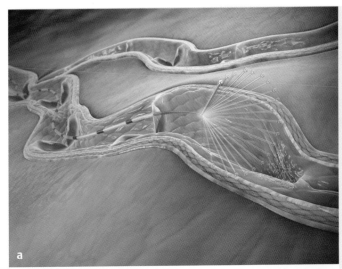

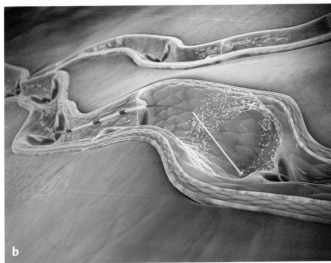

Fig. 10.5 (a) Rotating wire tip of the ClariVein device causes mechanical damage to the endothelium of the diseased vein. **(b)** Liquid sclerosant simultaneously released with wire rotation results in simultaneous chemical damage to the endothelium of the diseased vein. (Reproduced with permission from Vascular Insights, LLC.)

primary varicose veins.[30] The procedure is typically associated with either no sensation or a vibration in the leg that is not uncomfortable. Mild pain can be caused when the wire snags on either the vein wall or a valve, which tends to occur when the wire is rotated without pullback.[23] When compared with RF ablation of the incompetent GSV, MOCA is associated with significant less postoperative pain, faster recovery, and earlier work resumption.[32]

Prospective studies for MOCA have demonstrated closure rates ranging from 87 to 97%,[24,25,26,27,28,29,30] with a 2-year study reporting a 96% occlusion rate.[28] A randomized controlled trial comparing MOCA with RF ablation demonstrated similar occlusion rates of 92% after 4 weeks.[30] Another randomized controlled trial (MARADONA) is currently comparing the anatomical and clinical success of MOCA versus RF ablation at 1-year postprocedure.[31]

10.3.5 Complications

No major complications such as DVT, pulmonary embolism, or nerve injury were observed with MOCA. Reported minor complications include ecchymosis, superficial thrombophlebitis, and hematomas at the puncture site.[6]

10.4 Cyanoacrylate Embolization/VenaSeal™ Sapheon Closure System

10.4.1 Overview

Cyanoacrylates are liquid adhesives that have been safely used in numerous medical applications including brain arteriovenous malformation embolization, retinal repair, and wound and tissue closure.[33] The VenaSeal™ Sapheon Closure System utilizes a proprietary cyanoacrylate formulation that is delivered endovenously to treat varicose veins.[34,35,36,37,38,39,40] Contraindications for Vena-Seal include hypersensitivity to cyanoacrylates, acute superficial thrombophlebitis, thrombophlebitis migrans, and acute sepsis. Safety in pregnant women and in pediatric patients has not been established.[34]

10.4.2 Mechanism of Action

The proprietary VenaSeal adhesive is n-butyl-2-cyanoacrylate based and formulated to increase viscosity, decrease the rate of polymerization, and result in a flexible adhesive end product. Cyanoacrylate polymerizes in a cascade reaction upon contact with blood, creating an adhesive bond. The formed adhesive halts blood flow through the vein and the adhesive is eventually encapsulated in a fibrosis reaction to establish chronic occlusion.[34,35]

10.4.3 VenaSeal™ Device and Technique

The VenaSeal™ delivery system components include a 5-Fr catheter with an effective length of 91 cm, a 7-Fr introducer with an effective length of 80 cm, a 5-Fr dilator with an effective length of 87 cm, an adhesive dispenser gun, dispenser tips with a length of 3.8 cm and an inner diameter of 1.5 mm, 3-mL syringes, and a 0.035-inch 180-cm J-tip guidewire.[34]

The vein to be treated is accessed distally with a micropuncture kit or equivalent under ultrasound guidance after administration of local anesthesia. For treatment of the incompetent GSV, the introducer/dilator system is advanced to the level of the SFJ over a guidewire under ultrasound guidance. The introducer tip is then positioned 5 cm distal (inferior) to the SFJ. Using a dispenser tip attached to one of the provided 3-mL syringes, the cyanoacrylate adhesive is drawn up from its vial

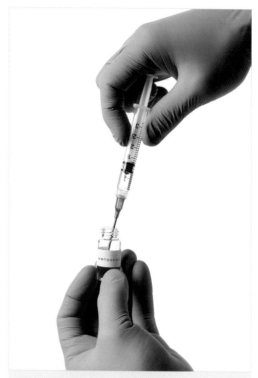

Fig. 10.6 VenaSeal adhesive being drawn up from vial. (Reproduced with permission from Medtronic.)

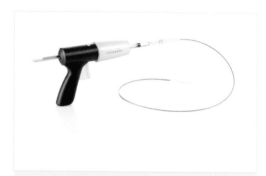

Fig. 10.7 Assembled VenaSeal delivery system with adhesive-containing syringe attached to catheter and dispenser gun. (Reproduced with permission from Medtronic.)

(▶ Fig. 10.6). The syringe containing cyanoacrylate is then connected to the VenaSeal catheter and its plunger end locked into the dispenser gun (▶ Fig. 10.7). The catheter is then primed by pulling the trigger of the dispenser gun. Each depression of the trigger delivers a controlled 0.10-mL amount of adhesive. The primed catheter is inserted into the introducer and advanced under ultrasound guidance until its tip is positioned 5 cm distal to the SFJ. The ultrasound probe is then turned transverse, placed just cephalad to the catheter tip, and pressure is applied to compress the GSV near the SFJ, sealing off venous outflow. While applying compression to the GSV, two injections of 0.10-mL adhesive are delivered at 5 and 6 cm distal to the SFJ. The introducer and catheter are then withdrawn by 3 cm while holding transverse compression for at least 3 minutes. Following this, 0.10 mL of adhesive is delivered every 3 cm along the vein to be treated while holding ultrasound compression just caudal to the previous injection for 30 seconds after each administration. Treatment is stopped 5 cm cephalad from the access site. Similar technique is performed for treatment of the incompetent SSV.[34,35]

Postprocedure use of compression stockings is not required, but some patients may benefit from compression depending on severity of disease. Neither tumescent anesthesia nor patient sedation is required.[36]

10.4.4 Outcomes

Three major studies have been performed, the First-In-Man feasibility study, the eSCOPE study, and the VeClose trial.[36,37,38] In the feasibility study, the 30-day occlusion rate was 97% and the 1-year occlusion rate was 92%.[36] In the eSCOPE study, 3-month occlusion rate was 94%.[38] The pivotal clinical study, VeClose, was a randomized trial of 222 subjects comparing VenaSeal™ CAE to RF ablation.[37] Tumescent anesthesia was used in the RF ablation group but not in the CAE group. Compression stockings were used in both groups to reduce bias. Three-month closure rates were 99% for CAE and 96% for RF ablation, proving noninferiority of CAE.[37] Patients did not wear compression stockings in either the feasibility or eSCOPE studies.[36,38]

10.4.5 Complications

In the VeClose trial comparing CAE and RF ablation, intraprocedural pain was self-rated by patients as mild and similar for both procedures. Less ecchymosis was present in the treated region at day 3 in the CAE group compared to the RF ablation group, presumably due to lack of tumescent anesthesia. Superficial thrombophlebitis was seen in 6% of the CAE group versus 3% of the RF ablation group.[37]

No major complications such as DVT, pulmonary embolism, or nerve damage were observed with CAE in any study.[36,37,38]

10.5 Investigative Nonthermal Ablation Techniques

Additional nonthermal ablation techniques exist, but these have limited published evidence thus far. The V-Block procedure consists of placement of a conic basket distal to the SFJ with or without endovenous infusion of liquid sclerotherapy. This procedure has only been performed in animal trials with promising results.[39] Laser-assisted foam sclerotherapy (LAFOS) utilizes a low-energy laser immediately preceding foam injection. The laser energy was sufficiency low that no tumescent anesthesia was necessary. In a pilot study of 50 subjects, 100% occlusion was seen.[40]

References

[1] Hoggan BL, Cameron AL, Maddern GJ. Systematic review of endovenous laser therapy versus surgery for the treatment of saphenous varicose veins. Ann Vasc Surg. 2009; 23(2):277–287

[2] Luebke T, Gawenda M, Heckenkamp J, Brunkwall J. Meta-analysis of endovenous radiofrequency obliteration of the great saphenous vein in primary varicosis. J Endovasc Ther. 2008; 15(2):213–223

[3] Mundy L, Merlin TL, Fitridge RA, Hiller JE. Systematic review of endovenous laser treatment for varicose veins. Br J Surg. 2005; 92(10):1189–1194

[4] Gloviczki P, Comerota AJ, Dalsing MC, et al. Society for Vascular Surgery, American Venous Forum. The care of patients with varicose veins and associated chronic venous diseases: clinical practice guidelines of the Society for Vascular Surgery and the American Venous Forum. J Vasc Surg. 2011; 53(5) suppl:2S–48S

[5] Pronk P, Gauw SA, Mooij MC, et al. Randomised controlled trial comparing sapheno-femoral ligation and stripping of the great saphenous vein with endovenous laser ablation (980 nm) using local tumescent anaesthesia: one year results. Eur J Vasc Endovasc Surg. 2010; 40(5):649–656

[6] Sadek M, Kabnick LS. Are non-tumescent ablation procedures ready to take over? Phlebology. 2014; 29(1) suppl:55–60

[7] King JT, O'Byrne M, Vasquez M, Wright D, VANISH-1 Investigator Group. Treatment of truncal incompetence and varicose veins with a single administration of a new polidocanol endovenous microfoam preparation improves symptoms and appearance. Eur J Vasc Endovasc Surg. 2015; 50(6):784–793

[8] Todd KL, III, Wright DI, VANISH-2 Investigator Group. The VANISH-2 study: a randomized, blinded, multicenter study to evaluate the efficacy and safety of polidocanol endovenous microfoam 0.5% and 1.0% compared with placebo for the treatment of saphenofemoral junction incompetence. Phlebology. 2014; 29(9):608–618

[9] Paty J, Turner-Bowker DM, Elash CA, Wright D. The VVSymQ® instrument: use of a new patient-reported outcome measure for assessment of varicose vein symptoms. Phlebology. 2016; 31:481–488

[10] Todd KL, III, Wright DI, VANISH-2 Investigator Group. Durability of treatment effect with polidocanol endovenous microfoam on varicose vein symptoms and appearance (VANISH-2). J Vasc Surg Venous Lymphat Disord. 2015; 3 (3):258–264.e1

[11] Carugo D, Ankrett DN, Zhao X, et al. Benefits of polidocanol endovenous microfoam (Varithena®) compared with physician-compounded foams. Phlebology. 2016; 31(4):283–295

[12] Carugo D, Ankrett DN, O'Byrne V, et al. A novel biomimetic analysis system for quantitative characterisation of sclerosing foams used for the treatment of varicose veins. J Mater Sci Mater Med. 2013; 24(6):1417–1423

[13] Regan JD, Gibson KD, Rush JE, Shortell CK, Hirsch SA, Wright DD. Clinical significance of cerebrovascular gas emboli during polidocanol endovenous ultra-low nitrogen microfoam ablation and correlation with magnetic resonance imaging in patients with right-to-left shunt. J Vasc Surg. 2011; 53 (1):131–137

[14] Wright DD, Gibson KD, Barclay J, Razumovsky A, Rush J, McCollum CN. High prevalence of right-to-left shunt in patients with symptomatic great saphenous incompetence and varicose veins. J Vasc Surg. 2010; 51(1):104–107

[15] Eckmann DM. Polidocanol for endovenous microfoam sclerosant therapy. Expert Opin Investig Drugs. 2009; 18(12):1919–1927

[16] Full prescribing information. Varithena. Available at: http://www.varithena.com/Portals/VarithenaHCP/Varithena_Full_-Prescribing_Information.pdf. Accessed June 20, 2015

[17] Rabe E, Pannier F, for the Guideline Group. Indications, contraindications and performance: European Guidelines for Sclerotherapy in Chronic Venous Disorders. Phlebology. 2014; 29(1) suppl:26–33

[18] Asciutto G, Lindblad B. Catheter-directed foam sclerotherapy treatment of saphenous vein incompetence. Vasa. 2012; 41 (2):120–124

[19] Williamsson C, Danielsson P, Smith L. Catheter-directed foam sclerotherapy for insufficiency of the great saphenous vein: occlusion rates and patient satisfaction after one year. Phlebology. 2013; 28(2):80–85

[20] Ceulen RP, Jagtman EA, Sommer A, Teule GJ, Schurink GW, Kemerink GJ. Blocking the saphenofemoral junction during ultrasound-guided foam sclerotherapy— assessment of a presumed safety-measure procedure. Eur J Vasc Endovasc Surg. 2010; 40(6):772–776

[21] van den Bos R, Arends L, Kockaert M, Neumann M, Nijsten T. Endovenous therapies of lower extremity varicosities: a meta-analysis. J Vasc Surg. 2009; 49(1):230–239

[22] van Eekeren RR, Hillebrands JL, van der Sloot K, de Vries JP, Zeebregts CJ, Reijnen MM. Histological observations one year after mechanochemical endovenous ablation of the great saphenous vein. J Endovasc Ther. 2014; 21(3):429–433

[23] Mueller RL, Raines JK. ClariVein mechanochemical ablation: background and procedural details. Vasc Endovascular Surg. 2013; 47(3):195–206

[24] Elias S, Raines JK. Mechanochemical tumescentless endovenous ablation: final results of the initial clinical trial. Phlebology. 2012; 27(2):67–72

[25] van Eekeren RR, Boersma D, Elias S, et al. Endovenous mechanochemical ablation of great saphenous vein incompetence using the ClariVein device: a safety study. J Endovasc Ther. 2011; 18(3):328–334

[26] Bishawi M, Bernstein R, Boter M, et al. Mechanochemical ablation in patients with chronic venous disease: a prospective multicenter report. Phlebology. 2014; 29(6):397–400

[27] Boersma D, van Eekeren RR, Werson DA, van der Waal RI, Reijnen MM, de Vries JP. Mechanochemical endovenous ablation of small saphenous vein insufficiency using the ClariVein(®) device: one-year results of a prospective series. Eur J Vasc Endovasc Surg. 2013; 45(3):299–303

[28] Elias S, Lam YL, Wittens CH. Mechanochemical ablation: status and results. Phlebology. 2013; 28 Suppl 1:10–14

[29] van Eekeren RR, Boersma D, Holewijn S, Werson DA, de Vries JP, Reijnen MM. Mechanochemical endovenous ablation for the treatment of great saphenous vein insufficiency. J Vasc Surg Venous Lymphat Disord. 2014; 2(3):282–288

[30] Bootun R, Lane T, Dharmarajah B, et al. Intra-procedural pain score in a randomised controlled trial comparing mechanochemical ablation to radiofrequency ablation: the Multicentre VenefitTM versus ClariVein® for varicose veins trial. Phlebology. 2016; 31(1):61–65

[31] van Eekeren RR, Boersma D, Holewijn S, et al. Mechanochemical endovenous Ablation versus RADiOfrequeNcy Ablation in the treatment of primary great saphenous vein incompetence (MARADONA): study protocol for a randomized controlled trial. Trials. 2014; 15:121

[32] van Eekeren RR, Boersma D, Konijn V, de Vries JP, Reijnen MM. Postoperative pain and early quality of life after radiofrequency ablation and mechanochemical endovenous ablation of incompetent great saphenous veins. J Vasc Surg. 2013; 57(2):445–450

[33] Spotnitz WD. History of tissue adhesives. In: Sierra D, Saltz R, eds. Surgical Adhesives and Sealants: Current Technology and Applications. Lancaster, PA: Technomic Publishing Company, Inc; 1996

[34] Venaseal Closure System Instructions for Use. Available at: http://www.accessdata.fda.gov/cdrh_docs/pdf14/P140018c.pdf. Accessed June 20, 2015

[35] Lawson J, Gauw S, van Vlijmen C, et al. Sapheon: the solution? Phlebology. 2013; 28 Suppl 1:2–9

[36] Almeida JI, Javier JJ, Mackay EG, Bautista C, Proebstle T. Cyanoacrylate glue great saphenous vein ablation: preliminary 180-day follow-up of a first-in-man feasibility study of a no-compression-no-local-anesthesia technique. J Vasc Surg. 2012; 55:297

[37] Morrison N, Gibson K, McEnroe S, et al. Randomized trial comparing cyanoacrylate embolization and radiofrequency ablation for incompetent great saphenous veins (VeClose). J Vasc Surg. 2015; 61(4):985–994

[38] Proebstle TM, Alm J, Rasmussen L, et al. The European multicenter study on cyanoacrylate embolization of refluxing great saphenous veins without tumescent anesthesia and without compression therapy. J Vasc Surg Venous Lymphat Disord. 2013; 1(1):101

[39] Farber A, Belenky A, Malikova M, et al. The evaluation of a novel technique to treat saphenous vein incompetence: preclinical animal study to examine safety and efficacy of a new vein occlusion device. Phlebology. 2014; 29(1):16–24

[40] Frullini A, Fortuna B. Laser assisted foam sclerotherapy (LAFOS): a new approach to the treatment of incompetent saphenous veins. Phlebologie. 2013; 66:51–54

Index